The Mustache That Walks Like A Man

By William Wayne Montgomery, M.D.

I.S.B.N. 0-8338-0215-4

Library Of Congress Catalog Card Number

95-075082

Marshall Jones Company

Publishers Since 1902

Manchester Center, Vermont

PRINTED IN THE UNITED STATES OF AMERICA

Dedicated To My Corpsmen.
Those Who Made It And Those Who Didn't.

Acknowledgement:

I would like to thank Ruth Ann Bergmann, a talented young writer who assisted with the manuscript. Other acknowledgements to Pam Turner, Julia E. Montgomery, Peggi F. Simmons and Craig A. Altschul for their assistance. And, of course, my lab, Charlie, for his companionship.

-W.W.M.

Preface

This book relates some of the thoughts, feelings, and experiences of a man, who as a young boy grew up in rural Vermont. A boy who became a country doctor, then a combat surgeon in the United States Marine Corps during the Korean War. It is not specifically written for medical personnel; therefore most medical terminology is either explained or omitted completely.

I have written this book so that those who are personally and professionally associated with me can better understand my personality, attributes and defects, related to having been a combat surgeon with the Marines during the Korean War.

-W.W.M.

Contents

Introduction

It seems that the natural order of things continue...

My plane, the one I am to take from Boston to New York, is one and a half hours late. I guess, in the grand scheme of things it is always the same, no matter what airport you are in anywhere in the world, nothing is ever on time.

I surrendered to my fate and settled down in the waiting area. After all the travelling I have done in my life, I've actually grown to enjoy waiting, watching and observing. Waiting around gives me the perfect opportunity to take part in my favorite pastime, watching the world go by. It seems to me no matter where I have gone, no matter where it was in the world, there was always something to watch, observe, enjoy or learn.

I began to drink in my surroundings as I glanced around the waiting area, taking in all the numerous smells, the tapestry of colors, the melodic blending of sounds as the people and machines synchronized together within this little world. I embraced the pure, dynamic ambience of this particular place. This one spot was so like a bee hive teeming with activity, bees buzzing all around me trying desperately to get from one place to another, from the ticket counter to the gate to catch their plane, to pick up their luggage, or to embrace their loved ones in greeting or farewell. The activity was intoxicating.

There were so many styles, so many different attitudes, demeanors, variations of dress, it could be said the blend of people I beheld before me embodied the true spirit of the American melting pot, citizens of the world. Different, but similar in so many ways.

My mind wondered touching ever so briefly on each person or group, contemplating their life histories, their relationships with one another, their reasons for being here at this particular time. Were they here to greet someone or to say goodbye? Were they here to fly off on the next plane for recreation or business? Were they excited, sad, or a little nervous? I could spend endless hours imagining the possibilities.

My eyes settled on one particular couple with their two children. I couldn't take my eyes off them. For the life of me, I couldn't understand why I found these people so fascinating. They weren't that unusual, except they were in Middle Eastern Dress. It dawned on me that my destination was the Middle East and soon I would be the one who stood out in their homeland. Perhaps I was studying them, trying to find a way I could blend in their country. I watched them on and off over the top of my newspaper, making sure I didn't make them uncomfortable, until the announcement came over the P.A. my flight was ready to board. I located my seat and happily found there wasn't going to be anyone seated next to me. Yes! No idle conversation to take part in. I could be quiet and think. This was turning into the beginning of a great trip.

I sank down into my seat and looked out the window. The sky was overcast and a few snowflakes began to drift down. The sight was beautiful. Offhandedly, I thought I would miss the snow while I was gone, but not the cold. My eyes began to close as the engine started and I began to relax. How long had it been since I really slept? Five? Six? Seven? It had been seven days, one whole week, since I had a good night's sleep. I was so glad the past week was behind me. Each day had been filled with so many hours of surgery, evaluating patients, hours of research, and preparing for this trip. It was a good feeling to know I would be away from the stressful existence at least for a while. I drifted away slowly and was asleep before we took off.

I awoke very slowly, feeling refreshed as we began circling New York for our landing. After we were on the ground, I grabbed my bags, left the Pan American area and headed for Saudi Arabia Airline. What I thought was going to be a short walk turned out to be the entire length of Kennedy International Airport. As I reached the Saudi Terminal, my arms were aching and I was short of breath. I realized I had packed too many things. It was over two hours before my flight was scheduled to take off. After talking to an airline employee I also realized I couldn't check in yet because I was going to be travelling with someone and I had the tickets, passports and visas for both of us.

As I stood, watching all the activity around me I barely noticed another airline employee approach and ask to see my ticket, explaining to me that it was standard policy that no one without a ticket be allowed in the area. Instantly his attitude toward me changed and he offered to check me in immediately. I declined, opting to wait for my companion. I figured it was the way I was dressed, in blue jeans and a sweater, not exactly everybody's idea of first class travel wear.

I placed my bags down in the middle of the lobby, sat down on the largest and attempted to keep myself entertained by watching the things around me. One quick look and I realized I was in the minority. Everyone else looked alike. The men had black beards and the women, the majority of them, were dressed in black with their faces covered. I had a strange feeling. I was struck by how uncomfortable I felt. I could sense, even though I could not see through their veils, that some of the women were watching me. I was usually the one doing the watching, but I was as different from them as they were from me.

An hour passed and I gave up watching and tried to keep myself occupied by repeatedly reading the same article, as every minute seemed to drag by, each slower than the last. I was uncomfortable. I contemplated going up to the V.I.P. Lounge, but the thought of lugging my bags up two flights of stairs suppressed my desire for more comfortable seating. I just shifted my weight, kept my eyes open for my travelling companion and sat.

Soon, before I even noticed, I was surrounded by about a dozen Middle eastern children, circling me like wild Indians around the wagon train. There was one difference: The Indians in the old west could not have been this loud.

My head began to throb, mostly from the children yelling, but also with concern. I had never met my contact person, my travel partner, Chris, before. I had no idea who or what to look for. Chris was also a doctor and, over the phone, he said he was tall, had dark hair and a mustache. He would be wearing blue jeans as well. Not a very detailed description, but I figured spotting another American in this area wouldn't be too difficult.

The children had grown tired of me and moved on to another waiting passenger. My headache was fading and my eyes were glued to the door at the entrance to the waiting area. As soon as Chris walked in, I knew it was him and I was more than glad to see him.

I greeted Chris and we took our places in line. Desert Shield was about to end in a few weeks, and if all did not go well, it would turn into Desert Storm. Chris and I were on our way to Saudi Arabia as experts in our fields. I, as a laryngologist, my specialty was diseases of the throat. He was a Pulmonologist, specializing in diseases of the lungs. As we stood waiting to board our plane I imagined that neither of us looked like experts in anything. Both of us in jeans and sweaters and looking like we hadn't slept in days.

About five minutes after we took our places in line, a ticket agent approached and offered to take our bags from where we were standing and check us in immediately. I gave thanks for first class travel and for the government that was footing the bill.

When everything was taken care of, Chris went off looking for the men's room. I passed the time by having my shoe's shined. I read the sign behind the chair and I climbed up and sat down. "Shine: $3.00 plus tip." Sounded reasonable to me. When I had settled in the chair, I put my feet in the metal footrest and said hello to the shoeshine man. No answer. Craving for some conversation I asked him, speaking louder than I had in the greeting, if he ever thought of what happened to the shoes he shined, where they travelled to, since he worked in an airport. The man looked up at me blankly and when I finished talking he said, "Me give good shine." Then he began to shine my shoes.

I was slightly surprised. I believe he hadn't been to school, at least in this country. I shrugged and looked out the window until the shine was completed. It was snowing harder than when I landed, coming down now like a white rainstorm. I wondered if the plane was going to take off. Chris joined me and we walked to the gate.

Shortly after we were seated, the pilot announced we were going through a de-icing process, which was quite apparent to those sitting in window seats because there was red liquid dripping down the outside of the windows. The storm had become a minor blizzard. It continued to fall as we sat in the plane on a snow-covered runway. It fell for many more hours.

When it finally stopped, the runways were plowed and we were ready to take off. We hadn't been anywhere yet, but we were extremely tired. As I drifted into a blissful rest, I was suddenly awakened by an announcement over the loud speaker. There was a cat on board and they wanted to know if someone would claim it because it was about to be taken off the plane. I hoped it wasn't black. To some people, black cats are good luck, but to me, on a plane that was just about to take off, it was a bad omen. I still don't know if the cat was black, I merely prayed it wasn't.

Finally, the plane raced down the runway, and I started to relax in my luxurious surroundings. The first class seats on this particular plane were truly fit for royalty.

The long flight was going smoothly and quietly until we were about an hour from arriving at Jeddah, Saudi Arabia, when all the Saudis changed into their native garb and prayed. Everyone in the first class cabin took part, except for some of the crew and Chris and I. It was an honor to observe another culture at prayer. I noticed what I thought was a clock on the ceiling and then determined it wasn't a clock at all, but a compass. When I asked, a flight attendant explained the passengers prayed in the direction of the compass because it was always pointed in the direction of Mecca.

We landed smoothly in Jeddah. It was wonderful to be on solid ground again. The absolute beauty of Jeddah struck a chord in me. I had known its seacoast was legendary, a true haven for SCUBA divers and a photographer's dream locale. I could see so many scenes that would make a great picture that I couldn't wait to get to my camera. Any thoughts of getting that "one" photo for the Pulitzer were dashed when a Saudi military person told me not to take pictures. I walked back to the gate and into the jet for the last leg of the trip.

We were soon airborne and shortly arrived at our final destination, Riyadh, the capital city of Saudi Arabia. It had been forty-eight hours since I had left Boston, two whole days without a shower or decent food. I think I had slept no more than a total of six hours on the trip. I was exhausted, and I felt like I was walking in a fog. Chris and I wandered slowly through the airport looking for our contact. Someone was supposed to meet us, but he was nowhere to be seen and we had no description.

Fed up and exhausted, I put my bag down where we stood and asked Chris where do we go now and what are we supposed to do. Chris began to look around. I stared at his face as he scanned the airport. slowly, a grin began to form around his mouth, then it turned into a full-fledged smile. He saw something!

"Look over there! Maybe that's our man," Chris yelled. I slowly stood and looked toward where he was pointing. I saw a short man holding a sign which read, "Riyadh Military Hospital". We ran over to the man and began to ask questions. Sure enough, he spoke English and explained he was to be our driver. I was never so happy to see a stranger before in my life. He said he had been waiting for us for many, many hours, but didn't say exactly how many. I had a feeling it hadn't been too long. We got the rest of our luggage and he drove us to our hotel.

Our lodging was to be the Intercontinental Hotel, which currently housed most military personnel and exiled rulers from Kuwait.

After I slept for what seemed like a nanosecond, Chris and I began to do what we had come here for. Over the next few days, we visited many hospitals and we never got enough sleep. It was the night of the third day before I could look forward to a good eight hour's rest. As I waited for sleep to come, I thought of how the native people seemed to be nervous and anxious. They had every right to be since no one really knew what Saddam Hussein's capabilities really were. I fell asleep thinking about the situation and the possibility of war...the best fodder for bad dreams.

I woke up with a start. It was a 4 a.m. and still dark. At first, I couldn't figure out what caused my abrupt awakening. I soon ruled out a bad dream. What woke me I could still hear. I heard it again and it sent shivers down my spine. In the distance was a loud speaker giving an announcement in Arabic. All I could think of was the war starting. A dozen questions went through my mind. Was it a raid? What was I supposed to do? I waited motionless, waiting for something to happen. There were no instructions in English and nothing happened. I waited and waited and finally fell back into a fitful sleep. I awoke the next morning feeling more tired than the day before and learned over breakfast that the announcement was nothing more than the first call to prayer for the Moslems.

Riyadh itself is an oasis sitting in the midst of a vast desert. Everything is modern. It is hard to believe that one mile from the city limits, the desert begins and goes on for what seems forever.

In the evening, we drove out beyond the city limits and saw a camel caravan in what I could only describe as a sea of sand. As we drove down the road, I wondered how these people survived in such an inhabitable place. I realized they survived much like their ancestors had for thousands of years before them, and hopefully, how their descendants will survive after them. Their lifestyles had changed little over the centuries. They have remained constant in an ever-changing world. All over the globe, change has come, everything modernizing, shifting more rapidly as each new day passed into the nest. Everywhere except here. Centuries passed, days passed. Yesterday is the same as today and today is the same as tomorrow. But, sadly I knew change was coming to this sandy oasis. And, soon. It was almost January 15, 1991. The day Desert Storm was scheduled to begin. The day when everything would change.

War was almost inevitable. The view of the barren desert before us suddenly shifted and gave way to a large number of soldiers hurrying about their duties in their desert uniforms of tan and gray. In some form, war was coming.

My thoughts turned abruptly back to another place, back to another time, forty years ago, back to another batch of soldiers. United States Marines, back years ago to...KOREA 1951-1952.

Chapter One

A DAY IN THE SUN

My eyes opened slowly as the crimson rays of the morning sun intruded upon my emotionless dreams. I sat upright with a jolt, realizing how my body was awake, but my mind still lingered in the misty landscape between dreams and reality. I gently rubbed the sleep from my eyes. I had slept long and hard, hour after hour drifting from dreams to nothingness and back again, but for all my sleep, my body felt sore and tired, as if the hours I had slept had only been minutes.

The dawning sun grew brighter, bathing my living quarters in an eerie reddish glow, its warming light pouring through a small eastward opening on the far wall of my bunker, slowly thawing the icy haze of sleep that still clung to my tired brain.

My mind cleared and grasped reality. It was time to get up. I reluctantly climbed out of the warm comfort of my sleeping bag and stared up at the roof of my bunker, willing my body to get going. I was startled as my ears detected the distant sound of artillery fire, not the expected sweet morning song of the birds. After all this time I still, halfheartedly, expected the cherished birds of Vermont to wake with me instead of enemy fire. Morning had come again to the 38th parallel on the western coast of a peninsula called Korea.

Emerging into the cool morning air I shivered, delighting in the chill. I knew that this would be that last time until tomorrow morning that I would actually be cool and comfortable. Putting off the day just a little longer in order to relish the moment, I searched my brain trying to remember the date.

"I know it's the beginning of the Summer of '52, which has already been too hot and too long for my taste. June, but June what? June 7th. It is June 7th, 1952. I counted backwards. I think it's a Saturday."

No one was ever really sure from one day to the next what day of the week it was. It didn't matter. Each day blended and disappeared into the next very similar day. When things got busy we sometimes misplaced days, even weeks, never knowing or caring. Other important facts, statistics, and matters clutter the brain. The day of the week soon becomes the last thing on your mind.

I heard the camp waking up, moving around outside, as the sun climbed higher into the sky. The light filled my bunker with a red-amber haze. Then the ubiquitous olive green began intruding from the corners of the room. I sighed and reached over to the foot of my drab green cot, grabbed my drab green uniform and began to pull it on over my drab green t-shirt and drab green shorts, then walked out into the glorious orange rays of sunlight.

My thoughts came together in one voice, "God, or someone, or something like God must exist. In the midst of all this killing and chaos, we find eternal beauty and miracles. If only people would pay more attention to what is good in the world and each other instead of what is bad."

I took a deep breath, inhaling as much of the peace as I could and wiggled my toes, thankful I had forgotten to put on my boots. My bare feet

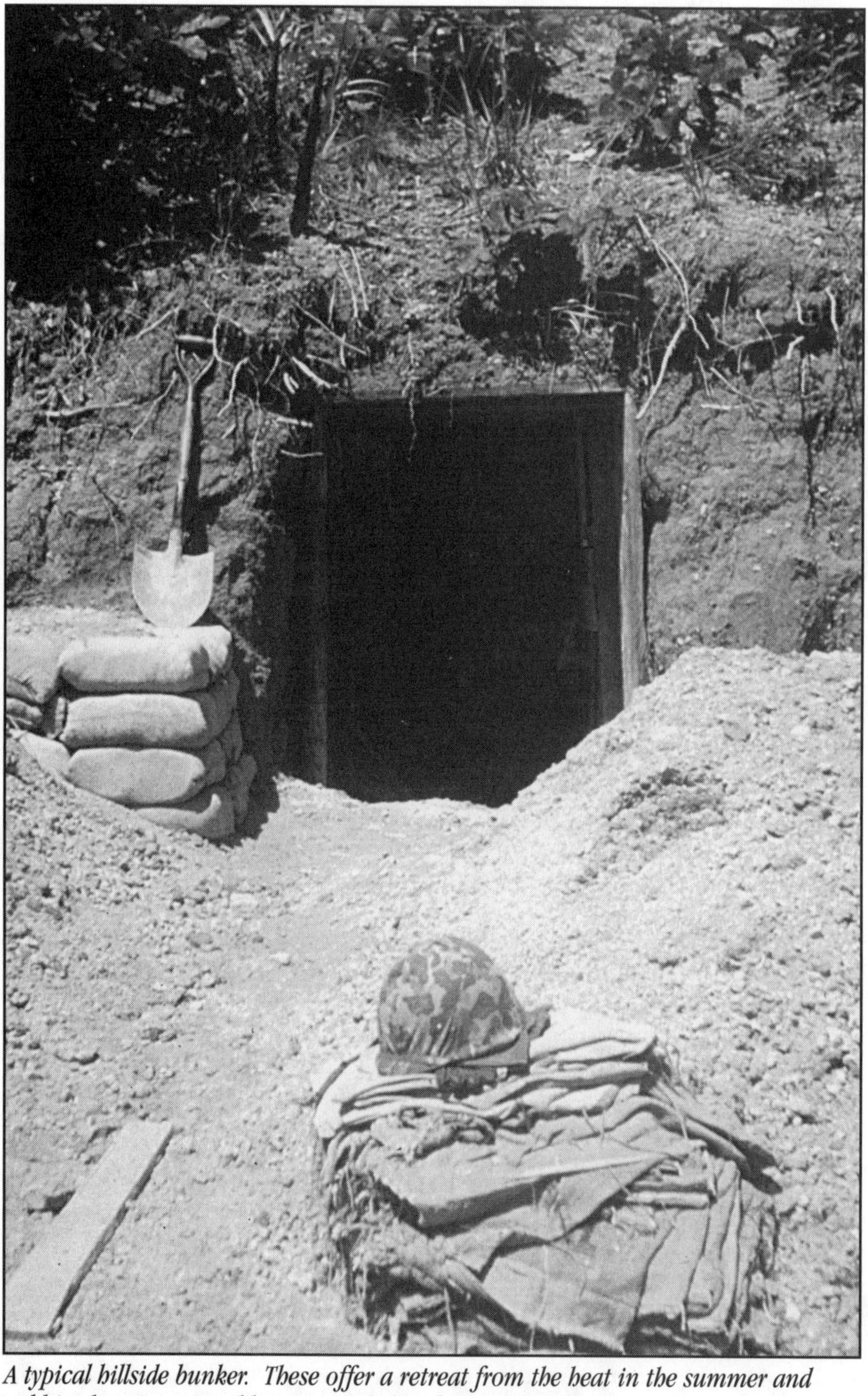

A typical hillside bunker. These offer a retreat from the heat in the summer and cold in the winter in addition to a shelter from enemy fire.

felt cool upon the hard packed sand in front of my bunker. I felt wonderful. I looked around, my eyes drinking in my surroundings, everything was being bathed in a bright orange glow, changing slowly, yielding to a burning amber and then the yellow gold of the daytime sun.

Our battalion was situated in a small valley surrounded by a few small 'mountains', which to my eyes resembled large hills rather than mountains. I was used to larger mounds of earth being called mountains, like the Green Mountains of Vermont, my home state, or the Adirondacks of New York, or the White Mountains of New Hampshire. The 'mountains' that surrounded us here weren't quite worthy of the description, as they were really only large hills, but everyday, small though they were, I was thankful for their protection and for the wonderful setting they provided for these beautiful sunrises.

As I stood and watched, the sounds of war, the distant rumble of artillery fire, faded quietly away. I stood there not moving for minutes; hours could have passed and I wouldn't have cared. All I cared about was what was in front of me, right in front of me, the sunrise. I didn't want this moment to end, the day to continue, the night to come.

But, the day had started and I had to get going too. I reluctantly began my morning stretches, like every day, and thought of what was on the day's schedule for me, what was in store for me. All I knew was it was inspection day. Like so many days that have come before, it was time again for routine sanitary inspections. Since the days lately had been so hot it was important that the battalion surgeon, me, and my corpsmen perform the inspections. Not a job I ever look forward to, especially on a hot summer's day but, it had to be done and I'm one of the ones who had to do it.

We inspected all the living facilities that housed the marines, from occupied houses and tents to bunkers and foxholes. Everything had to be inspected for health hazards.

The morning progressed slowly as the sun climbed higher in the clear blue sky, drowning everything below in an intolerable heat. My two corpsmen, Jim Haskins and Howard Smith, Corporal Wagner and I went from bunker to bunker, from inspection site to inspection site each blending into the next as we searched for health hazards, seeing if the marines had kept their insect and rat populations to the bare minimum; most of them had, who wouldn't?

On our inspections we also made sure they all had an adequate drinking water supply; in this heat it was a number one priority. They kept their water in lister bags for easy access. Most marines, after having had so many lectures on sanitary conditions, disposed of their garbage and waste correctly and tried desperately to keep clean while living in the dirt, but always the smells lingered. So many odors, each distinct and sickening, decayed together into an almost sweet nauseating smell, each playing on a different nerve. At times all you could do was smell, no other sense you had could function. Luckily today, despite the heat, I could see straight and the smell was unpleasant but bearable.

During the course of the morning as my thirst grew, along with my comrades, I thought of how easy it could be to construct an outdoor shower. At least there could be some relief from this sweltering heat. My dream would drift into practicality and reality. What could be a better target for a sniper than a bare assed marine out in the open taking a shower. My mouth felt as if I had swallowed all the dust in Western Korea, my only hope of rescue from the heat slowly rested upon getting something, anything, to wet my parched mouth. I was so thirsty. How I wished to be waist deep in a cool running river back in Vermont, drinking lemonade, being back home, cool and comfortable.

The morning crept slowly into the afternoon, as the sun reached midheaven and my comrades and I reached George Company Headquarters, our task of routine inspections was nearly complete. Each one of us were now drenched in sweat. It looked like the heavens had open on us and given us the cooling shower we had been praying for. Everything we had on was saturated with perspiration.

We went from bunker to bunker through George Company inspecting each and paying our respects to the men. As we approached bunker after bunker, one thought screamed continuously inside my mind, it would be great to have something cold to drink. I knew that some of these bunkers had homemade 'refrigerators' called floorpits. These floorpits were only small holes about two feet square and two feet deep dug into the dirt floor and covered by anything flat that could be found, usually a plank of wood. These 'refrigerators' kept things pretty cold, cold enough on a hot summer day like today. Bunker after bunker my thought and prayer for something cold to drink slowly became a whisper, defeated; no one offered us a drink, cold or warm.

We finally made it to the battalion officer's bunker, tired, hot, sweaty and thirsty. The officer in charge, Lt. John Hughes was busy on the field phone so I decided to ask the sergeant for something to drink. As he handed me, and the others, luke warm Coca-Colas, he explained that there wasn't any beer around these days. I didn't care the moment the Coke passed through my lips and I tasted the refreshing sweetness of the cool brown liquid. I believed this was the elixir of life, nothing ever tasted that good, and I believed nothing ever would again. I was satisfied down to my very core. We all sat down onto wooden crates and sipped what was left of our Cokes in silence, treasuring each and every wet, thirst-quenching sip.

Suddenly, bursting through our reverie, Lt. Hughes bellowed from across the tent. His phone conversation became louder and more animated with each passing second. From what I could gather the lieutenant was in contact with the patrol leader of a scout party which had been in enemy territory for most of the night. Lt. Hughes' voice rose higher in excitement, there was a definite sound of genuine concern in his voice. The look on his face slowly softened and turned cold.

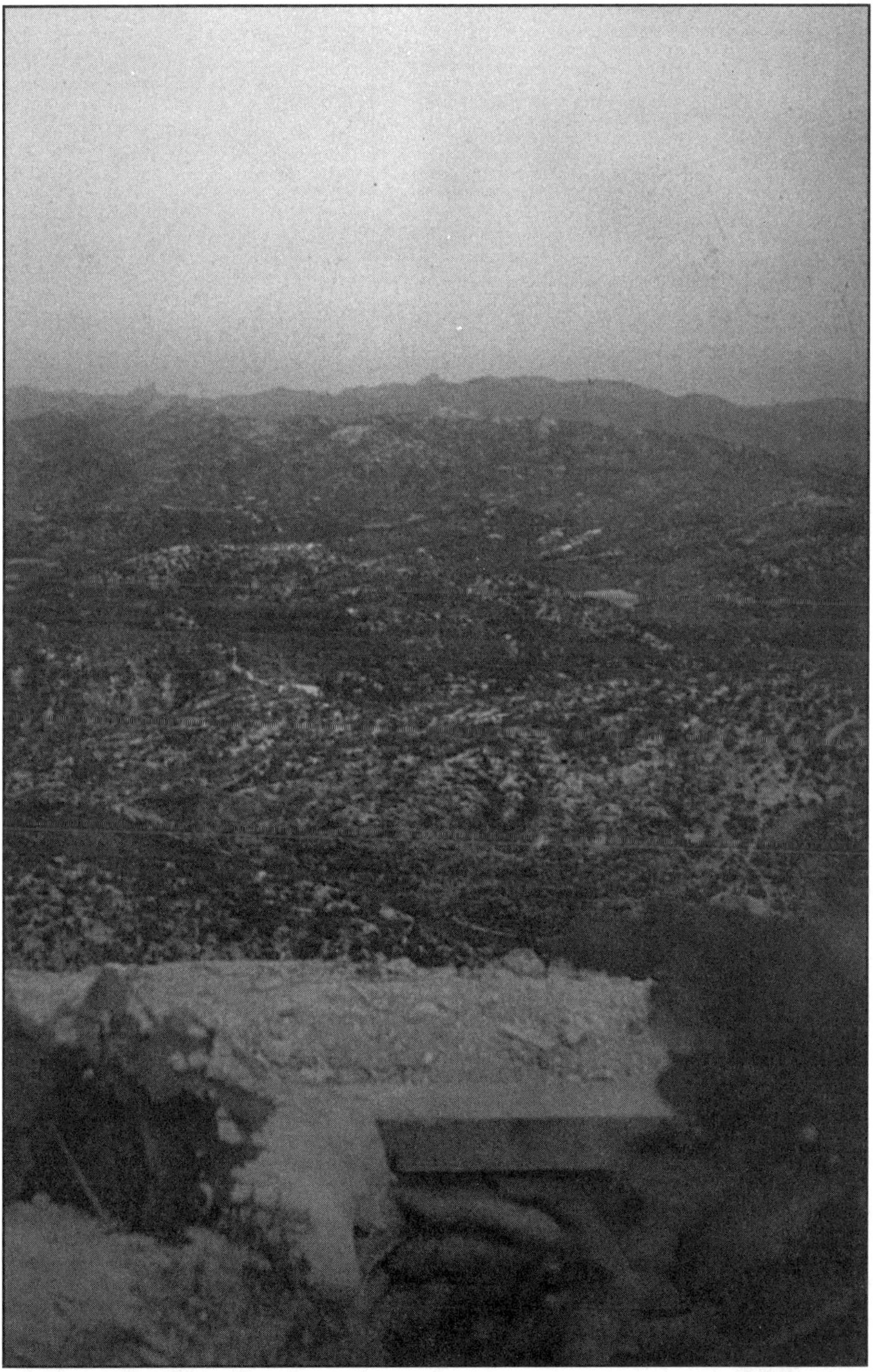

A view of enemy territory from a foxhole. Field glasses and patience would most often reveal enemy troops.

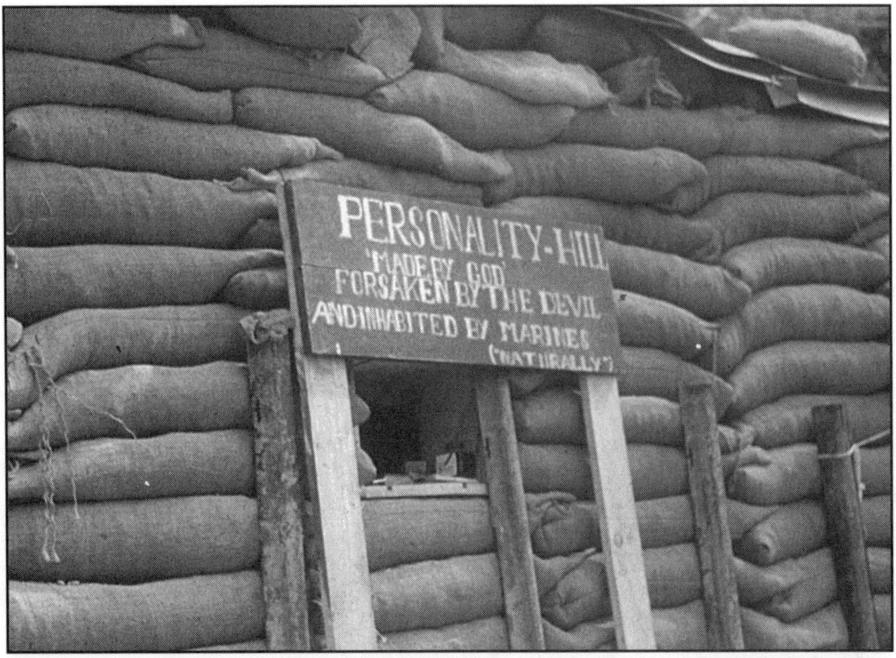

A bunker on the front line. The sign reads: "Personality Hill – Made by God, Forsaken by the Devil, and inhabited by Marines (Naturally)". Note the defects in the sandbags made by shrapnel.

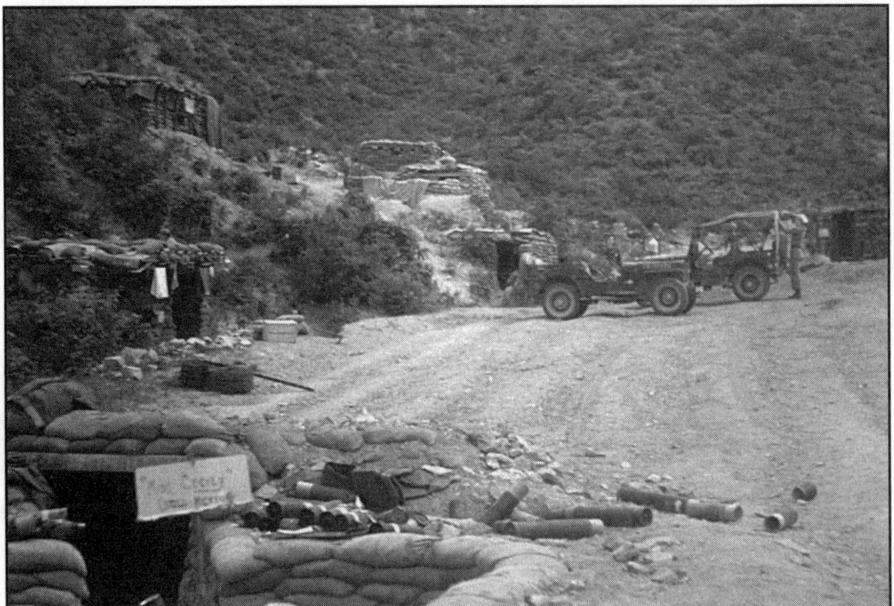

One of our mortar companies the morning after a busy night of combat.

"Okay, okay. Stay where you are. I'll get help to you. What!? How many? Oh, Christ! Son of a bitch! Do your best for them. I'll get help to you soon, as soon as I possibly can. Hang in there."

The lieutenant signed off with the slamming of the receiver, shook his head and then cranked the field phone initiating a call. Quickly he barked a code name, I knew then he had called in the whirlybirds. My heart sank, this was serious. The whirlybirds were the small helicopters with the 'bulletproof' plastic bubble in front and the two casket-like body containers on each side of the landing gear. These helicopters could carry only two wounded out of an area at one a time, but they could evacuate an amazingly large number of wounded, flying in and quickly flying out, in a short period of time. If the copters could get to the patrol they would probably be okay.

As I tipped the soda bottle back and the last drop of cola tricked down my throat we heard the distant, familiar churning of the helicopters. The sound seemed to shake the very ground beneath us as they landed. As soon as the helicopters touched the ground Lt. Hughes was up and out of the bunker to talk to the pilot. After he left the bunker we sat in silence waiting to find out what was going on. Following a long conversation, longer than I would have expected for an emergency, Lt. Hughes returned, his face painted a picture of unguarded anger, his cheeks red with emotion. The lieutenant was quiet until he was completely inside the bunker and had sat down on an empty wooden crate. His head, hanging low, was supported in his right hand. A low sigh escaped from his lips as he looked up and spoke to us.

"Man! I've got 17 marines out there on patrol. They were ambushed and are still under some fire. God only knows how many are bad hit. The patrol leader sounds really shook up. Their corpsman is wounded. I've got to get medical aid to them and get them evacuated pronto. The pilot out there said he has strict orders to stay south of the front line. Which means he'll go nowhere near those men. I've got to get them out of there."

Lt. Hughes looked straight at me and Jim Haskins, one of my corpsmen. He eyes silently asked for help. He didn't have to say a word.

"I'll go. Who the hell is going with me?" I asked jumping up. My mind asking myself, "What are you doing?" I didn't know what I was doing, I didn't even know I was going to volunteer until I found myself standing and the words pouring out of my mouth, proclaiming my intentions. I just knew I had to go. I found myself continuing, "I am not very familiar with that territory and if they are still under fire, I want to know what I'm getting myself into."

I did know the area, somewhat. I had been in this vicinity since the winter before. I just wanted everything covered,including my own ass. Slowly Jim stood up and volunteered to go with me. That meant Jim , Corp. Wagner, the driver, and I were going in there after the crippled patrol. Lt. Hughes broke into a grateful grin, pleased he was getting

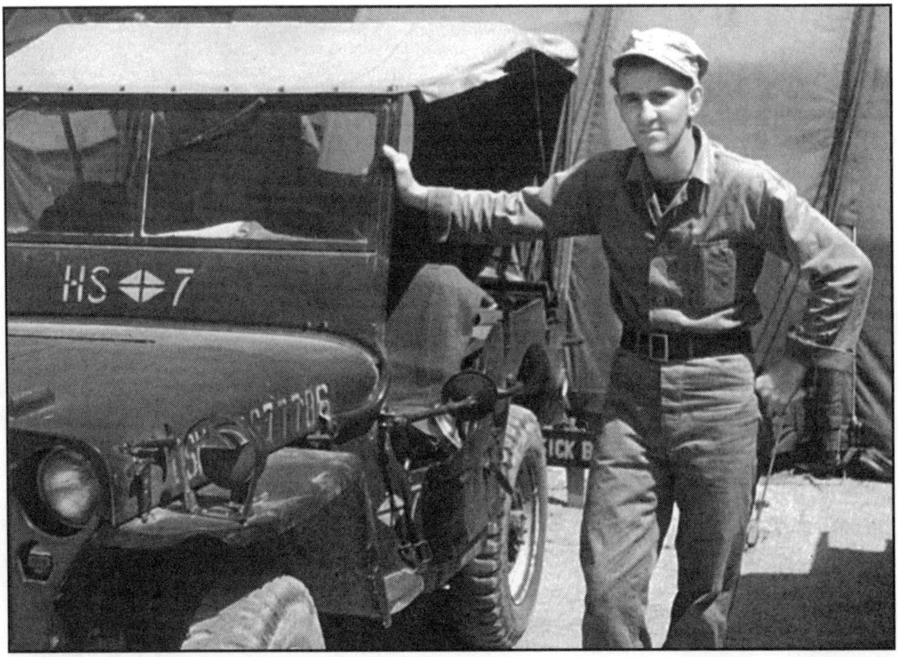

Corporal Wagner and his jeep.

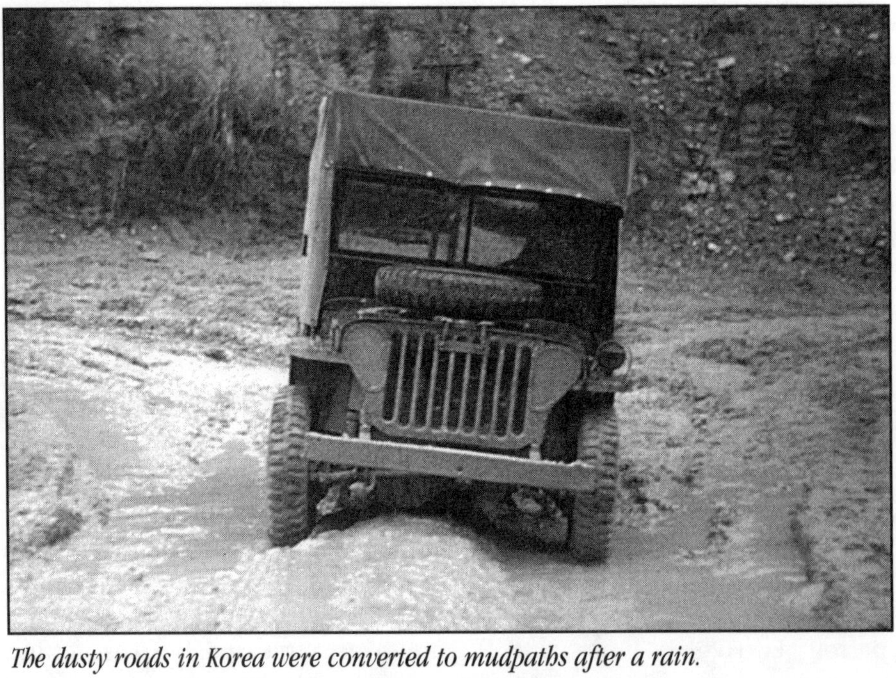

The dusty roads in Korea were converted to mudpaths after a rain.

someone to the patrol, and quickly showed us where they were on the field map.

"I'll call in artillery to keep the gooks in their caves for a while and I'll send an officer along with you." Lt. Hughes said, smiling reassuringly. Why is he so happy? I thought to myself. Because he wasn't going was the answer. Jim, Wagner and I sort of saluted as we hurried out of the bunker. This was definitely no longer a routine day.

Corporal Wagner started the engine as soon as he jumped into the jeep. Jim and I, close behind, jumped in and we took off. We were soon traveling down the main dirt road at 'breakneck speed', almost twenty-five miles per hour. I now understood why, as a general rule, we never traveled faster than twenty miles per hour. The road was too rough and we kicked up too much dust. Soon a dustcloud was starting to form. I'm sure we would have been engulfed in a full- fledged dust storm if it weren't for the fact that we had rain the day before. The thunderstorm had brought some relief from the heat and thankfully had packed down some of the dirt. Unfortunately, it also left in it's wake some treacherous water-filled pot holes. Wagner was doing his best to maneuver around the "pond-sized" holes but we were kicking up so much dust that by the time we turned off the main road we were completely surrounded by a brown cloud. The dirt was everywhere, inside everything, in places I didn't even know existed. As we progressed higher and higher up the slope the narrow road became more and more impassable. The path was more like a series of potholes than a road and we became hopelessly mired in the mud. Jim and I got out of the jeep and pushed it as Wagner tried to direct us and the jeep in the right direction. The temperature rose and the sun baked the dirt and mud onto our skin. We couldn't move the jeep. So far this mission was starting out with a bad finish. We couldn't even get started.

We struggled, pushed, cursed, and sweated. The jeep didn't move. Then, right when we started to lose hope, a friendly voice came from behind us.

"You won't be able to go much farther up the path in the jeep. You might as well stop trying."

It was a marine lieutenant who introduced himself as Frank Andrews. He was going to be our guide. The mission hadn't ended before it began; we were going on. We decided to leave Corp. Wagner with the jeep, and Jim, Frank and I, would go ahead on foot. We proceeded single file. Frank led the way, I was second and Jim was in the rear. The sky had turned a picture-postcard blue and there wasn't a cloud in sight. There was no breeze, no comforting coolness. The heat was unbearable, sweat flowing out of every pore, dripping into my eyes faster than I could wipe it away. My eyes burned and my sunglasses kept slipping from their position on the bridge of my nose. I was slowly becoming more and more miserable. The world was still, there was no sound except for the crunching of our boots on the dry earth and an occasional whisper from one of us. Frank stopped suddenly, turned to Jim and me and whispered:

"Stay a couple of paces behind me and try to follow in my steps. There are quite a few mines out here; most of them, I think, are in the rice paddies, not in the path. I just want to make sure you don't wander off into a rice paddy and get yourself blown up. Besides, we may run into some 'gooks' and I'm better at spotting them than you are."

Okay. That sounded right to me. He really didn't have to say that. It was a foregone conclusion that I was going to follow him anyway. I had no wish to make my own way in this territory.

"Where do you figure the patrol is, from here?" I asked Frank in a hushed whisper. Frank slowed his pace and answered quietly, not turning around,

"A little over a mile and to the right. See over there?" Frank raised his hand and pointed over to the right of us.

"See that rise we are coming to and the peak of that small hill beyond it? Look where that artillery shell just exploded."

I nodded. Frank continued, picking up his pace, "Well, they are on the western slope of that hill. We call it "Outpost White."

Suddenly a burp gun belched in the distance. I didn't think it came from the direction in which Frank had been pointing. I wasn't sure where it came from.

The familiar churn of helicopters approaching from the rear caused me to turn and look up. There were two large army choppers flying southeast. I knew immediately that they belonged to the truce delegation from Munsan, for those were the only army helicopters in our sector. I looked towards Frank, ahead of me, and commented, "It must be another ten minute peace meeting at Panmunjon." I paused, then asked, "By the way, Frank, where is Panmunjon from here?"

"Two miles due West, Doc. You can see it from the top of the next rise. Hold on when we reach the top of this rise," Frank warned, slowing his pace. "We'd better survey the land ahead of us. There could be 'googlies' out there, ya know." I heard Jim utter an oath under his breath. None of us wanted to meet with the enemy. No way! Frank continued, looking back at Jim and me over his shoulder, "We're in enemy territory now. Don't either of you forget it for a second."

I looked back at Jim; he had the same look on his face as I'm sure I did. How did Frank think we could forget that we were in enemy territory. We knew where we were. We weren't about to forget that minor detail.

I did as I was instructed, following to the letter, staying a couple feet behind Frank. I kept pace with him and watched my feet, keeping my steps exactly in his tracks. My head ached, as if my helmet were on too tight. No chance to loosen it now. I looked up at Frank's back. I could see the sweat stains, turning the drab olive color of his field jacket to a wet dark green. I imagined he had two grenades in the inside pockets of his jacket, like most marines do in this type of situation. I myself, being the doctor, didn't have room for grenades inside my field jacket. Instead,

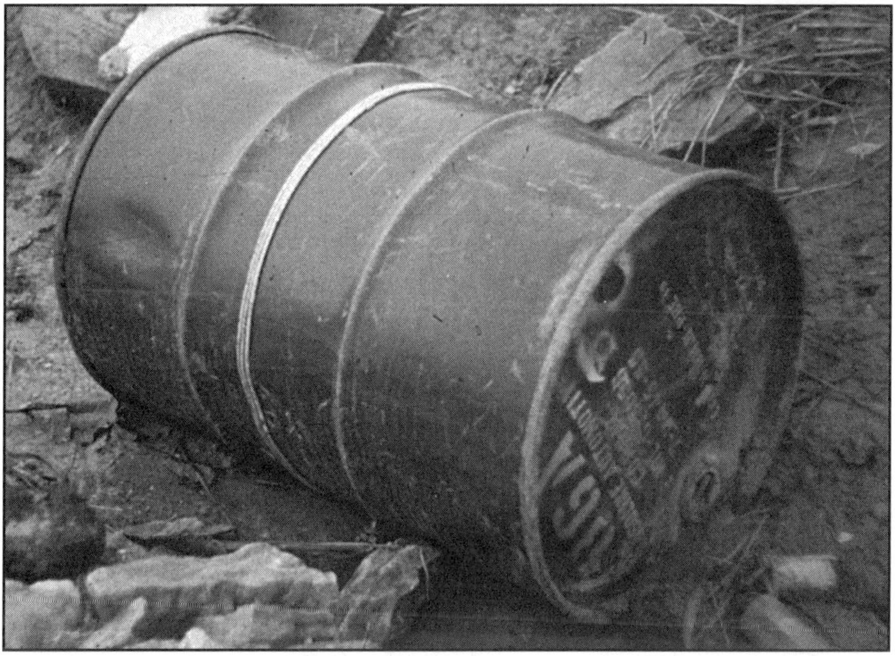

A napalm booby trap washed into sight after a heavy downpour. The trip wire would set off an incendiary grenade which in turn would ignite the jellied gasoline contained in the drum. The resultant explosion can wipe out an entire company. napalm is also used as fuel for the flame thrower.

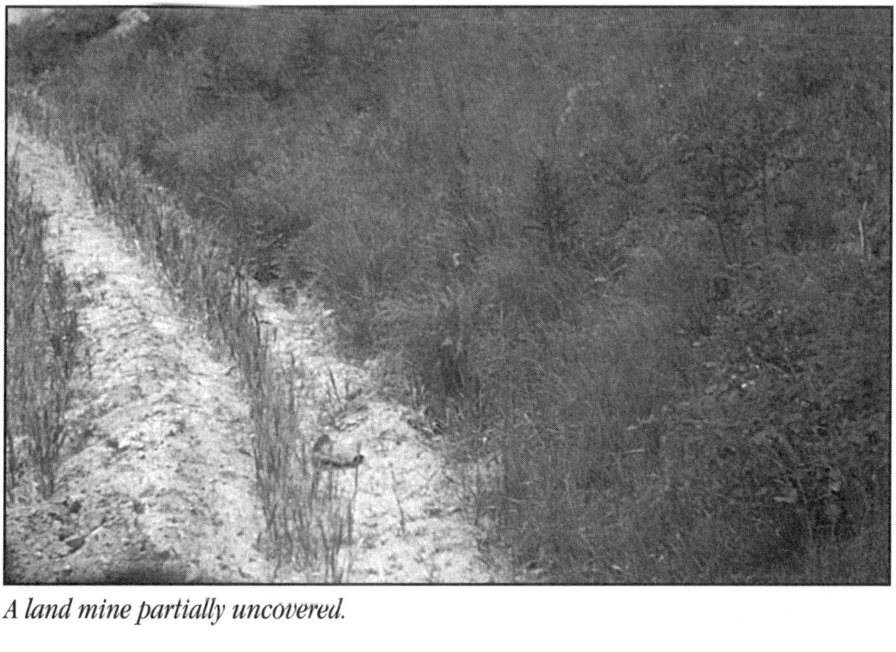

A land mine partially uncovered.

I carried several tourniquets I had made out of inner tubing, morphine tartrate syrettes and a couple of field dressings. I also carried my field medical kit on my back and at my side the standard issue, "we-can-assemble-it-blindfolded", 45 automatic service pistol. A thought suddenly bugged me as it scratched its way into my brain; the other reason for carrying this gun, suicide. We had all vowed not to be taken prisoner. I wondered if I had the guts to destroy my body with this gun. My mind came back to what I was doing. I studied Frank's tracks, putting my shoes carefully into the footprints he left in his wake. Lt. Frank Andrews was, I realized, a typical marine officer, posture perfect and ready to lay down his life for his country, a true blue, or drab green, marine. My eyes focused on my boondockers, then to Franks boots in front of me, back to my feet and then the ground beneath me. All I was thinking of was where I was walking, not where I had been or where I was going to, just where I was walking at that moment. One step in front of the other, one foot beyond the last. That was all. Step, step, step, that was all that mattered. Except.... for the sweat dripping slowly down my back. Suddenly a chill ran up my spine and halted at the base of my neck, marching out its cold cadence down through my core. My soul shivered.

I shook it off and focused on Frank's boots in front of me, concentrating on the sound they made as they crunched in the dirt. I was mesmerized. The sweat that was pouring down my face barely bothered me. It was if I was entranced, hypnotized. We reached the top of the rise and stopped. As I looked around I could see clearly into the next valley. The view was clear for about a hundred miles. As we stood there in silence, for a few minutes I forgot about the enemy out in front of us. It was like time had disappeared. There was no war going on, there was only peace.

It was time to move on so we started to descend the hill. I turned to say something to Jim, who was a few paces behind me, when heaven and earth along with hell and sky shattered apart. The world splintered into a million sharp pieces. The air roared around me, rushing in and out of my ears at a deafening speed.

I was flying through the air, hurtling to nowhere, totally out of control. Then, I hit the ground. All I could sense was the smell, the stench of an outhouse, human feces. I had landed on my back in a rice paddy. It was common practice to use human feces for fertilizing rice paddies. The odor enveloped me, and took over my whole being. All I could comprehend at that moment was the stench.

Slowly, gratefully, my other senses returned. I felt slightly dizzy and I heard a thunderous roar in both of my ears. I felt for broken bones, nothing. As I methodically moved and sat up, I realized my sunglasses were shattered and there was a burning sensation on the right side of my face. I had been hit! My hands were filthy. Without touching I could tell I was bleeding. I tasted blood. My right eye burned, my sight disappeared into a reddish blur. Blood was dripping down over my right eye, down my face and into my mouth. The deafening roar in my head and dizziness were clearing rapidly. I tried shaking my head in an effort to clear the noise. This sent shooting pains through my face, my wounds burning like wildfire. I stopped moving. The blood was pouring more rapidly, it moved faster and faster down my face and neck and onto my jacket. I listened to the sounds in front of us slowly become silent. I looked behind me, Jim was lying in a ditch taking cover. He had been far enough back that he hadn't been hit. Taking a deep breath I yelled over to him,

"Hey, Jim! Look at my face. Is it cut up bad?" I was startled. My yell was nothing more than a harsh whisper. It was hoarse and guttural. My voice had become strangely alien to me.

"No," Jim answered, his voice was shaky and scared. "I - I don't think so, Doc. Christ, Doc! This is bad, real bad. We'll never get out of here alive. We're going to die here. Right here in this damned rice paddy! We're going to die Doc, aren't we? What the hell happened Doc? What happened?" He looked as scared as I felt. I knew there was no way he was going to move. He waited for me to answer him. He waited for anyone to answer him. I tried to think of something reassuring to say.

I quickly answered. "I don't know what hit us, Jim. If it was a mortar shell there'll probably be another one soon." Not a very reassuring statement.

Suddenly, we were both startled. There was a moan from the other side of the summit. It was Frank. I've heard men cry out before, when they are wounded. I knew from the sound Frank had made his injuries were serious. I yelled to Jim to stay put and I cried out to Frank, my voice weakening, its volume becoming less audible, "Hold on, Frank! I'll be right there."

"Please Doc, hurry! It hurts so much. I can't stand it much longer...I..." Frank's voice faded, he was becoming weaker and weaker by the second. I had to get to him, fast. What about the mines? I questioned myself. Oh, boy! What was I going to do now?

"Doc, Doc! Look!" Jim yelped from behind me.

I turned and looked behind me to see what he was pointing at. About a yard away from where Jim was lying was a large piece of flesh, my stomach reeled. It had to have been Frank's. My mind screamed, I had to get to Frank.

I felt around me, my field pack was gone. I knew that there was more than a good chance that there were mines between Frank and me, and between Jim and me. I could have bet the farm in Vermont that there were.

Jim wasn't hurt and he wasn't going anywhere. I had to get to Frank. Thousands of questions went whizzing through my mind, all at once. Would I be able to get to Frank without getting blown up, too? Probably.

Frank was hurt badly, dying. With my field pack gone, where could I get some supplies? Jim's field medical pack! How far was it to where Jim was? About 15 feet. If I did get there, would I be able to help him? I'm a doctor, that's what I'm trained to do. What was my third grade teacher' s name? What was I thinking? I can't remember that now. How far was it to Frank? About 30 feet. How could I still be in one piece when I was only a couple of feet behind Frank? God only knows. Did I have it in me to go across the mine-laden paddy to get to Frank? I took a deep breath, secured my helmet and started crawling on my belly, towards Jim. I reached him in several minutes, minutes that seemed hours long.

"Mrs. McCarthy," I whispered. "That was her name." How I had loved the third grade.

"What?" Jim looked puzzled.

"Nothing," I explained. " I need your field medical pack."

Jim nodded and handed me his pack. As I started crawling over towards Frank, Jim warned,

"Be careful."

I nodded. I slowly inched my way back up the rise toward the spot where the explosion had occurred. I reached the summit, looked over it, and saw Frank about fifteen feet down the other side. He was lying partly on the path and partly in the rice paddy. His face was covered with blood. It had to have been a mine. It had to have been.

I knew now that I was crawling in an enemy mind field. How was I going to proceed? I had no bayonet to probe for them and I wouldn't really know how to use it if I did. I realized the grim reality that the enemy could be waiting out there for me. My only weapon was my 45 automatic. My brain felt like it started to sweat. My mind reeled. I had to get to Frank, no matter what. My body didn't move, no matter how much my mind begged, I couldn't move an inch. Frank screamed in pain again. My body began to obey my mind and I advanced slowly towards Frank. I didn't explode. I thought to myself, if I was going to get blown up I might as well start crawling and get it over with. So, with held breath, I started I to crawl. I moved faster and faster towards Frank, my mind

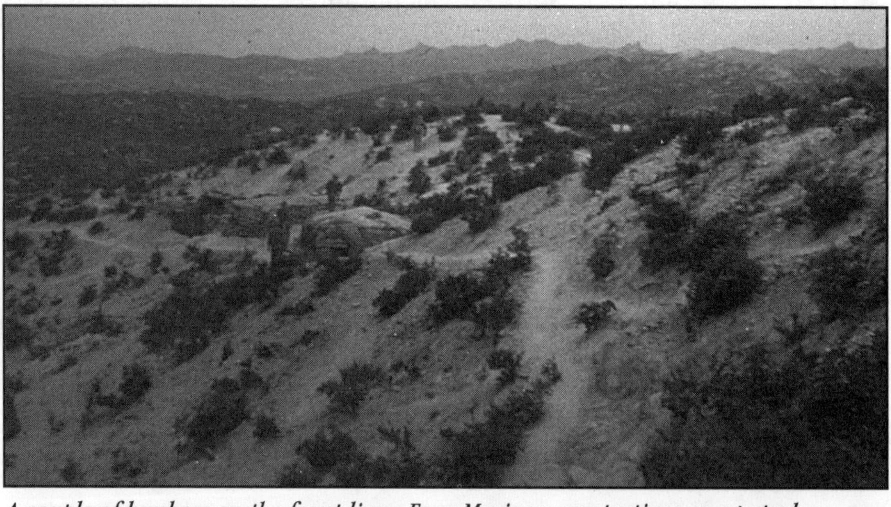

A couple of bunkers on the front line. Four Marines are starting on a patrol. Can you find them?

was blank except for the task in front of me, to get to Frank in one piece. I no longer could sense anything except my own concentration. Then, after an eternity, I reached the bottom of the slope and Frank.

Frank's eyes flickered open as I started to inspect his facial wounds. He took a ragged breath and pleaded, "Ungh. Doc, thank God you're here. Do something! Anything! I'm in terrible pain. Shoot me. Kill me if you have to! Just make the pain stop!"

"It's okay, Frank. It's going to be okay," I whispered, as reassuring as I could be. "We are all going to get out of this alive."

Frank's manner seemed to calm at my words. I knew we were going to get out of there. At least I hoped I knew. I fumbled through my pocket for a morphine tartrate syrette and attempted to inject the morphine intravenously. The attempt at injection failed, his veins had collapsed. He was in shock. Frank was still now, too still. Then he spoke in a hushed whisper,

"My leg is gone, isn't it?"

I didn't answer him. I looked down to what used to be his right leg. The morphine fell from my now shaking hands. His femoral artery was rhythmically spurting bright crimson blood. Without thinking I reached into the right inside pocket of my jacket and pulled out a strip of rubber innertubing. I quickly applied the innertubing as a tourniquet. The bleeding didn't stop. I applied a second tourniquet, slowly the blood stopped. I made a silent prayer in thanks and continued my arduous task.

I reached into the other side of my jacket, into my left pocket, took out another morphine syrette and attempted, in vain, to administer it intravenously. I knew there was no time to expose his shoulder muscle so, I injected the syrette right through his shirt. Soon, Frank's breathing calmed. He was feeling less pain; that or he was semiconscious. I sighed and looked closer at his facial wounds. They were mostly superficial and had, for the most part, stopped bleeding. I decided I didn't need to touch them. I dressed his right hand which had, at closer inspection, been cut pretty badly. Slowly, as I dressed his hand, I realized how much I hurt. Feeling was coming back. The adrenaline, which had been pumping through my system at full speed, started to wear off. Everything I felt hit me all at once. My face began to feel like it was on fire. My temples throbbed. I noticed the blood dripping into my eyes and it began to annoy me all over again. I waited, not thinking, just feeling.

Frank came to about ten minutes later, I think. I had lost all track of time. Frank seemed to be in much less pain. I was grateful for that. Frank questioned me again about his leg and I told him it was gone. He was silent, we both were. Frank fell back into a sleep.

WHOOSH! I nearly jumped out of my skin. It was artillery shells passing directly over our heads. I covered Frank with my own body and listened. I soon realized they were from our own artillery and were landing in enemy territory just ahead of us.

They were firing to keep the enemy down while we were in trouble.

Relief washed over me as I straightened up. They knew we were in trouble and where we were. This was a small comfort, but a well welcomed one.

I checked Frank's pulse, it was coming back fairly strong. What to do now, I asked myself. My gut feeling was to stay there and wait until someone came to get us. Deep down I knew that Frank was in too bad shape, emotionally and physically, to risk waiting for help for very long. I had to go get help, fast.

"Hey Frank," I said, shaking Frank gently. Frank roused. I continued, "I'm going to go for help. I don't think it would be too easy on you or me if I tried to haul you all the way back to the front line."

"Okay Doc," Frank replied in a hushed whisper. He moved nothing except his mouth. "Go ahead, I'll be all right," he continued," But you better get that damned copter from battalion HQ to come out here, fast. Even if you have to force the pilot's asses on to the copter with that thing on your belt you call a gun." Frank chuckled, which sent him into a coughing spell that racked his already weak body. I smiled. What a man he was. Still joking around. After Frank's coughs subsided and I knew he was going to be okay, at least for the time being, I took a deep breath and started out.

I had no bayonet to feel my way, so I began to crawl my way over the treacherous ground I traveled just minutes ago. I silently hoped, no, prayed, that I remembered where I had crawled before, where the ground was safe. Shells were reeling over my head. My brain was jumping rapidly from one idea to the next. By the time I had reached the point on the field where I knew that there were no more mines my mind was on overload. I had done more thinking in that fifteen minute crawl than I could normally do in five hours. My brain felt like it was oozing out of my ears, my emotions had disappeared, I felt nothing. That thought scared me more than any mine explosion ever could. I stopped, then continued crawling. I finally came to the level where Jim was lying. I called out to him and told him that I was going back for help and not to move because the area was loaded with mines. He agreed, with no argument. He wasn't going anywhere.

I continued to crawl. I thought I could crawl forever and never get out of this place. I crawled for about thirty yards, far enough so I could not be seen from the other side of the hill and far enough to where I was fairly certain there were no more mines. I stood up and ran like a bat out of hell until I got back to the jeep.

Wagner was still there, thank God. Good ole Wagner. He had gotten the jeep out of the mud with the help, I assume, of a Marine sergeant who was sitting beside him talking on the field phone. Wagner, who was the first one to see me, got out of the jeep and headed towards me.

"Geesh Doc, we heard the explosion. What the hell happened?" Wagner asked as he reached me. "Look at your face. Are you all right? Does it hurt?"

"I'm okay. Frank stepped on a mine," I gasped. "The googlies were waiting and they opened up on us. Jim's still taking cover by the path."

Wagner led me over to the jeep and let me catch my breath. The marine sergeant explained to me that he had already called for assistance via the lieutenant at the battalion. This I'm sure accounted for the shells going overhead while I was crawling. Soon, after my breathing returned to almost normal, we heard the welcome whirl of a helicopter. Faster than I could focus, the helicopter came into sight, flew directly over us, then landed next to where I was. The pilot looked at me, smiled and extended his head back as a questioning gesture. He pointed to his own face and then to mine. I can just imagine how awful my face looked covered with blood. I gave him an okay sign to tell him I was all right and pointed in the direction of where Frank and Jim were. The pilot nodded, waved and took off after my two friends.

Within a few minutes the copter had rescued both Frank and Jim. Two more helicopters appeared and went after the stricken patrol we were sent to rescue. While we waited for the rest of the men to be rescued, a 'four point two' mortar squad appeared, set up and pounded the enemy for a while to keep them real quiet while the helicopters were flying. These helicopters went back and forth and back and forth until the whole patrol was on safe, friendly ground.

I took inventory of myself. I looked down at my field jacket, there were tears from the shrapnel. My flack jacket had most likely saved my life. I vowed then and there to never complain about it again, at least not out loud.

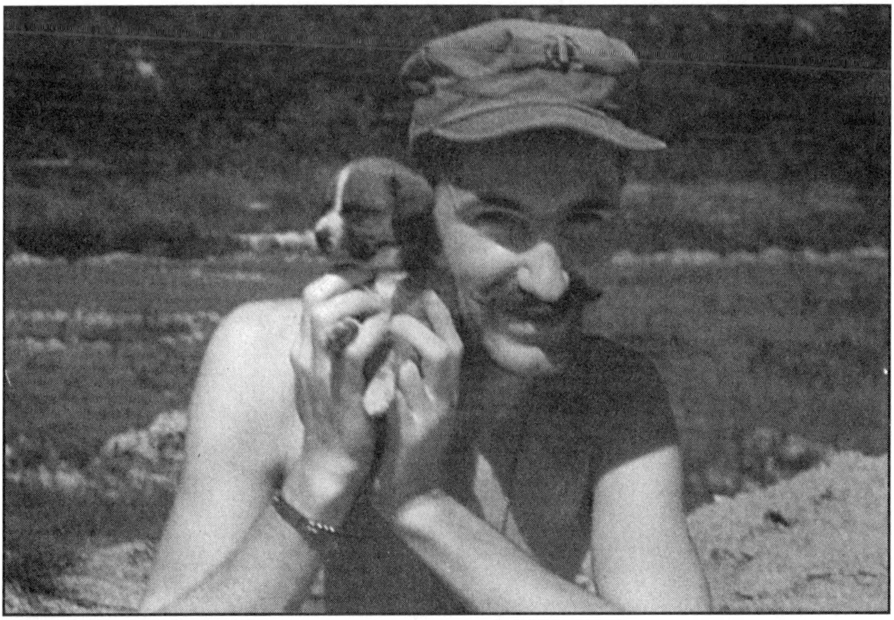

My little dog Georgie.

The world around me started to tip and I began to feel woozy. The whole experience suddenly hit me full force with a good, hard slap across my head. Wagner sensed I was feeling the effects of my trial and helped me into the jeep, drove back to the battalion and then subsequently to a regimental aid station. My whole body throbbed with fatigue and pain. My wounds were dressed and a corpsman gave me a penicillin and tetanus shot. I felt no pain from the shots, just an all over, brain soaking, fiery ache that existed in every cell of my being. As I waited to be released some one told me that Frank had made it back to the M.A.S.H. level and from there was evacuated to the hospital ship U.S.S. Haven, off the shore at Inchon. He was in good hands now and I knew Jim was okay, too. I breathed a sigh of relief, and lay down on the cot for a little rest.

I had rested for about an hour and I was starting to feel better so I decided to walk, slowly, over to the colonel's tent. As usual, as soon as I walked in he started to make me a straight up martini with an olive; I gratefully accepted. Over drinks, I related to the colonel all of the details of the incident. I asked him, when I was finished, if he would try to abort the telegram to my family stating that I had been wounded. He promised he would try everything in his power to do so, but from the look on his face I knew he had little hope of doing so. My heart sank. I didn't want them to worry about me. I decided to write to them as soon as I could. My letter wouldn't take the sting out of the hours that they would be wondering how wounded I was, but they would know straight from me that I was okay.

The colonel insisted on my going back to the M.A.S.H. level saying, "You made me go, Doc, when I took a slug in my thigh."

I agreed to go back to M.A.S.H. level, hesitantly. I was in no mood to argue. Wagner drove me back to "A" Medical Company (M.A.S.H. unit) where I was to stay overnight. By this time the pain was getting worse and I wanted some relief. The offering of a little sedation was welcomed. I rejoiced when Commander McLaughlin, the navy doctor who took care of me, gave me permission to go back to my unit the next day.

Every muscle screamed out in protest as I eased back upon the wobbly cot inside the M.A.S.H. unit tent. Before I could even stop it, a low moan escaped from between my clenched teeth. No one heard it though, its whisper lost among the other groans and moans filling the tent.

"At least I can get a good night's sleep here," I silently said to myself, more to convince my tired mind than an actual statement of fact.

As I waited there in the darkness for sleep, a flash of loneliness, more painful and frightening than anything that had happened to me in the last 24 hours, stabbed viciously at my heart.

I wanted to be home.

Home.

I just wanted to be...home.

All that had happened to me, since I came to these alien shores, hit me with such force, I felt my heart break. I had witnessed too much, seen too many grievous scenes, been witness to too many young lives ruined or cut short within a blink of an eye.

In a moment, everything can be altered. The powers shift.

Nothing is constant except change. Suddenly I felt an acute loss of my youth, my friends, my family, my home, my heart and my dreams.

"What is happening?" My brain questioned silently.

"No one knows, do they?" I asked no one...anyone.

"I am truly alone."

No answer, only silence.

SILENCE.

"Hey wait a minute, Buddy. What kind of thinking is that?" A voice screamed loudly in my ear.

I jumped and looked all around into the darkness that surrounded me. No one was there. I waited. Then, it dawned on me that voice had come from inside my own head.

"This kind of thinking just isn't healthy." The voice whispered.

Deep down inside I agreed. I had to think of something, anything.

As I laid there on the cot, I looked up above me through the darkness, up to the highest point of the tent and focused. Beyond I knew there were stars, bright and beautiful. There were stars just like the ones I watched in the night sky at home, maybe even some of the same ones I'd see at another time of the year. There were even stars behind a cloudy sky. The stars were always there.

I didn't have to see them, I knew it. With that one thought, a sense of calm returned. Was it the sedative finally kicking in or my realization? I didn't know. What I did know was that it was going to be okay. Everything would be okay.

I sighed slowly and closed my eyes, surrendering fully to the calming effects of the sedative. I drifted into a dreamless sleep. There would be another time to dream, other places to think, to search, when it wouldn't be so painful and my heart wouldn't be quite so heavy.

It was mid-morning when I walked back into my camp, back to my own regiment. The feeling, I can not adequately put into words, it was almost complete, pure happiness. I was so glad to be returning to the same old grind and to my little dog, Georgie. He had been a loyal companion to me ever since I had found him and kept him safe from being lunch for some of the locals. It felt as if I was almost home, almost.

The days moved slowly by. My mind occasionally drifted to the memories of what had happened to me, but I tried not to dwell too much on the past. The future is what I found myself thinking of more often than anything. I realized that it only took a fraction of a second to change your life. Frank had lost a leg and probably the use of his right hand in a blink of an eye. This ended his career as a marine. How would he adjust? How would I if I were severely wounded? I thought of my own wounds and remembered that, at the time, it didn't hurt too much and fear is usually the farthest thing from your mind, until afterwards. I came to realize that the events of June 7, 1952 gave me a new, better perspective as a marine combat surgeon. I felt that I could now relate better to the many wounded I would face and treat in the upcoming days and months.

The future I came to understand, is uncertain. War is never routine. I promised myself nothing would be the same again. I would enjoy every minute of every day. I would at least try.

Chapter Two

CREATURE AND OTHERS

I awoke in the dark solitude of night just before dawn, clutching my ears to make the endless sound go away. My head was buzzing, my ears were ringing. Each noise joined in a frightful harmony which screamed its chorus down through to my very soul. My mind pleaded for silence or at least some distance from the advancing enemy fire. The sounds of war had never left for a moment. One somehow slept through it only to awake when the rumble of outgoing artillery and the incoming whine and blast of return fire got closer and closer together or the small arms fire became louder and clearer. It had been six weeks since my close call on June 7th. My wounds had since healed, but my soul was still bruised, my nerves still frayed and my mind still tired. I am not sure if I was the same man I was before June the 7th. Somehow the 45 automatic pistol attached to my webbed belt, the carbine slung over my shoulder and the security of my flack jacket gave me comfort. I was again at ease with my lot as a combat marine doctor. It was time to get up off my ass and start the day.

The early morning sun was hovering over the rolling hills as we made our way from the 11th to the 5th battalion in our crackerbox ambulance. My two sidekicks, my personal corpsmen, HM1 Beauchamp and HM2 Rector were in the rear of the truck, poking their heads through the opening between the cab and the back. Corp. Wagner was next to me in the front, driving. The air smelled clean and fresh. The signs were promising that the day was going to get hotter, but there was a gentle breeze. We were all in good spirits. Our conversation changed quickly from one topic to the next. The questions most prevalent in all of our minds was when was the next push going to be, how were the peace talks going, what was going on back in the States?

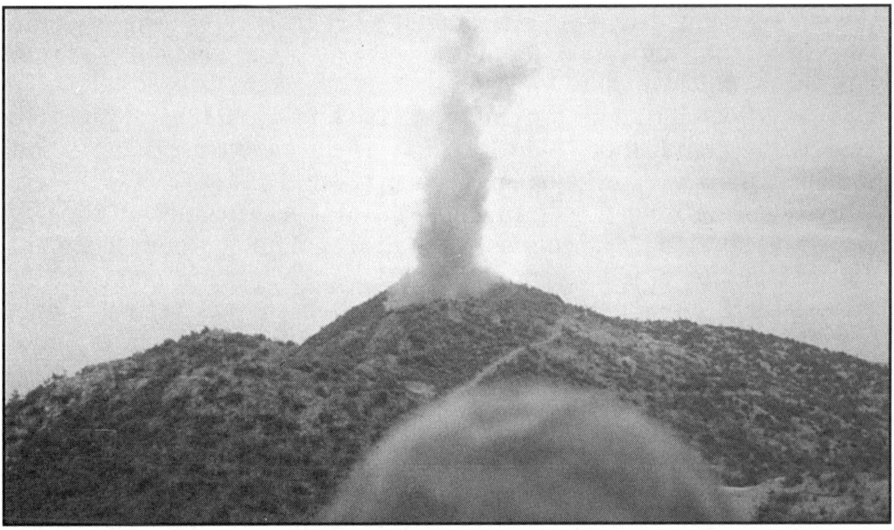

Noise and more noise. A photograph taken from a foxhole. The enemy shells were getting too close and it was time to find another hill and a new foxhole.

Suddenly all conversation stopped as if a part of us knew something was going to happen. A short piercing whine preceded the deafening blast. An incoming shell had landed near us on the side of the road. I reacted rather violently and hit my head on the roof of the vehicle. Shrapnel fragments whined by, some hitting the sides of the already dented ambulance, but none of us had been hit. None of the shell fragments had penetrated the steel of the ambulance. Then a second shell exploded, much closer and louder than the first. Wagner stopped the vehicle and we all reflexively dove from the vehicle into the roadside ditch facedown in the dirt.

I remember thinking, "Should I crawl under the ambulance?"

"Bad idea," part of me answered, "The gas tank could explode!"

I was really scared, for this was just too soon after having licked my wounds. I was "shook". I don't have any real good definition of shook. It's something you could get over, not like battle fatigue or shell shock. Shook is probably a temporary decompensation. I began to shake terribly. I was scared, for sure, really shook a pure feeling of complete fear which was something I had never felt before, and that terrified me even more. Somehow I had to get control of myself and not be a disgrace in front of my corpsmen and driver. I knew deep down that if I let my emotions fly now I might not ever be able to control them again. I pleaded to an unknown force.

The noise around me became louder, but strangely enough, my brain started to quiet. My more logical side started to take over. Suddenly I was able to turn off my left brain and put my mind in a blank state. Despite the chaos around me a peaceful calm washed over me and bathed me in tranquil serenity. I knew that I would come through the war. I would survive.

My mind calmed, letting itself wander away from this place. My mind concentrated on another time, another place where I knew all was right with the world. My mind took me away to a place where I had always felt safe. I floated back to my childhood, back to when I was 9 years old, back at my grandfather's side listening to the gentle plodding of our horsedrawn buggy slowly making its way down a dirt covered road with a strip of spring green grass growing in the middle. The muffled clip-clop sound was soothing. The sounds of the nearby shelling slowly faded into a welcoming fog of indifference.

I was there sitting next to Grandfather Potter. He was just as I remembered him, smiling down at me, making me feel like I was the most important person in the world. He had to have been about 70, his fringe of white hair blew gently in the wind as we headed farther away from town. I felt the cool breeze upon my skin and sighed. Potter, as I always called him, was speaking softly about his days as a professional baseball player. I don't know how many times I had heard this story, but at this moment I knew I didn't want the tale to end, I wanted him to keep talking forever. Potter obliged and I closed my eyes and listened, soaking up everything he was saying. Peace was all around me. Tom, the horse, neighed quietly, I could hear the trees rustle in the wind, the smell of the fresh country air and feel it's gentle breeze on my skin. I could hear the Robin's songs calling for rain mixed with the sound of a cricket's aria drifting by from a near by meadow. Even the distinct smell of horse manure, so different from a cow's, was a welcomed experience for my senses.

The buggy pitched as the horse jumped and twitched. My eyes suddenly flew open. There was an automobile coming at us from down the road. Tom had always been afraid of cars. He soon settled down, but the spell had been broken.

Things were fading and my vision was becoming blurred around the edges. The beautiful sounds of the birds were mixing with the harsh sounds of artillery fire. I looked at my grandfather. I wanted to memorize him, everything about him, the way he laughed, the way he smiled, everything, I never wanted to forget anything about him.

The sounds of the shells became louder, I could no longer hear what my grandfather was saying. I didn't want to come back to reality. It was too dark and unpleasant out here in the big world. I reached out to him, he turned and smiled his great big grin. My mouth opened and I tried to speak, but he couldn't hear me. A shell passed over head, he was fading, I could barely see his face. I didn't want him to go - not yet. "Grandfather!" He was completely gone in a flash of light as an enemy shell exploded nearby.

As I laid there, my forehead pressed into the ground beneath me, I tried to recapture my dream, my youth, but it all eluded me, just beyond my grasp, its solace slipped through my fingers. My mind raced as the shells kept roaring around me and the icy fear began to return, its cold apprehension creeping into me. I had to stop it. I had to force my mind to think of something else.

Soon my thoughts were back to my childhood again and in the town of West Rutland, Vermont, back to someone I thought I had forgotten but who came to my rescue now and pulled me into the past, "Creature" Lamphere, and the day he blew out the windows in all the houses of his neighborhood. Now that was a blast to remember.

Creature was one of the true geniuses who grew up in my small home town of West Rutland, Vermont. I always looked up to him for his genius and keen, albeit slightly strange, or perhaps deranged mind. It must have been his weird brain and bizarre activities that earned him his nickname and made him a legend at only 17. Although big for his age, he was quite normal looking, but oddly quiet and expressionless. You always knew he was thinking, but you could never tell what. He left a tantalizing trail of excitement for a youngster's imagination to follow.

At the time Creature's father was one of the only people in town with any money to throw around, which probably accounts for the reason Creature never ended up in the County House of Correction, for some of his escapades were truly wicked. His genius was demonstrated through electronics at which he was an expert. Of course, his car was electrified, but not in the usual sense. There was a button on the dashboard which he could push and deliver a 12 volt shock to anyone who touched the car. Well, this must not have been quite enough to thrill him so his next endeavor was to build a 1:1 scale model of an electric chair. It took some time to perfect. This time period mysteriously coincided with the strange disappearance of all the cats in the neighborhood.

One day he was ready to try it out on a larger species so he went in search of the perfect victim, who ended up being a kid named "Fat Fish". The first part of his name came from his appearance and the second from his intelligence, or lack thereof. I can't remember his real name. I guess Creature figured this was the only guy in town dumb enough to let himself be strapped into the chair. After a few jolts of electricity "Fat" was jumping around in the electric chair like his namesake in a skillet. He managed to break loose, finally, and ran sizzling up Clarendon Avenue to tell his mother.

Things didn't go so well for Creature for some time after that. The news made the front page of our local paper, the Rutland Herald, and Creature's mother was pretty rough on him. As a matter of fact, she carried out the punishment a little too long and he became quite upset with her and started scheming again.

Mrs. Lamphere had the only Franklin Coupe around, a beautiful 1927 model. She kept it well polished and when she wasn't driving, she parked it safely in the barn away from the damaging elements. Creature got himself a saw and must have spent a considerable amount of time sawing the beams under the floor of the garage about half way through. When she drove in the next day, her beautiful Franklin coupe went crashing down through to the next level. She didn't get hurt, but she was some mad!

He was grounded again, but I'm sure he used the time to plan his next venture, which was to rig mirrors up on top of his house facing the long causeway which led from the outskirts of town. As soon as a car came around the bend on this stretch of Route 4 in the afternoon, Creature's mirrors would reflect the rays of the sun directly into their windshields. Fortunately no one had a serious accident. Creature had to appear in Court for that one though, and remained real quiet for a long while.

One day Creature's parents decided to cut down a very large elm tree in their front yard. They left a stump which was too high for a seat and too low for a lawn table. This bothered Creature. He spent endless hours working on that stump. Chainsaws had not been invented. He used axes, wedges, saws and the like but made no headway. Elm is a very hard wood and the grain is interlocked so that splitting it is nearly impossible.

Finally, Creature began drilling holes in the stump with a one inch diameter drill bit which was about a foot long. This went on for at least a week. One Saturday morning, Creature got up at 5AM when no one was around and set to work on his project. Creature had stolen some dynamite from the Marble Company. Evidently he had read up on dynamite in one of his books. He put the sticks down in the holes he had drilled and attached dynamite caps and wiring. He then covered the stump with a foot of mud which he had prepared the night before. At 5:31 AM, the stump was blown away along with every window in the neighborhood that faced it. No one was hurt except Creature's rear end. He nearly went off to the County House of Correction for that one.

Even though Creature was about seven years older than I and in high school we became fast friends soon after we first met, almost certainly because he found out that I was good at building things. He needed an assistant. I couldn't resist the excitement. I felt like I was the apprentice to Dr. Frankenstein.

Our first project together was a full scale glider, with two cockpits, that we were going to fly at the first sign of spring. Creature already had the kit, we just had to put it together. After many cold winter months building the glider in the upstairs part of Creature's barn, the day had come to fly our wonderful "bird". His father agreed to tow the glider to the top of the town skipper slide which the CCC and the WPA had built for the children of the town.

This was a very unique area and I am sorry that it isn't here today for they constructed a highway across it. In order to explain all this, I have to tell you that the town of West Rutland is surrounded by mountains except for a pass on the east and west sides. The skipper slide was probably at least 100 feet wide and more than 1/2 mile long. Skippers were particular to West Rutland. They are made by attaching and fixing barrel staves under the rear end of a large plank, 1-1/2 by 4 feet, and a row of

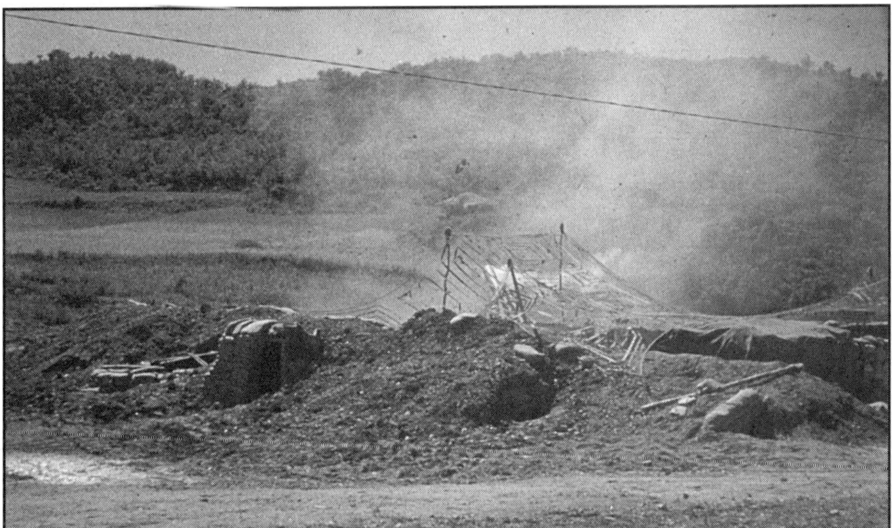

Returning fire with a well-camouflaged roving 155 Howitzer.

barrel staves on a swivel under the front. A rope attached to each side of the front barrel staves was used for steering. The rope was placed under a cross piece of wood in the front. That piece of wood extended out on each side to support the boots. The skipper was somewhat like a mini-bobsled and the steering mechanism was fairly effective, at least sufficiently so that you could travel down the length of this slide more than half the time without skidding sideways and taking a rather nasty tumble in the snow which resulted each winter in a few broken arms and legs.

As we approached the top of the slide, Creature told his Dad he could leave, then he and I prepared the "flying machine" for its maiden flight. The excitement was unforgettable. All my insides were jumping up and down in eager anticipation. We finally got the glider turned around on the top of the skipper slide, after what seemed like endless attempts. Creature got in the front cockpit, I then climbed into the back cockpit and we were ready to go. With a lurch we were headed down the steep slide. Half way down we were off, airborne. I never had felt so alive just gliding through the air, flying. I always had dreams of flying, but dreams didn't compare to the real thing. We drifted down slowly into the valley below and on to the high school football field. I soon realized, as the earth came rising up to great us, neither Creature or I knew how to land this thing. We had known a little about how to fly the glider, just what we had learned in library books, but we never read on how to land it. My joyous feeling of flying turn quickly into a overwhelming fear of crashing as we collided with the earth. No pain, no feeling, just stillness.

Nothing was broken I was sure. I just sat there and let the stillness envelope me. Time went by as I laid there, not wanting to move. There was no sound, not a bird, not a voice not even the breeze through the trees. The silence ruptured instantaneously into a pulsating explosion of chaos and confusion. I looked up into the sky above the high school and saw two saber jets flying overhead towards the north.

I had returned to the present. The jets hadn't been flying over Vermont, they were here, where I was, in Korea baking under the hot sun. They were there to lend support to the marines ahead of us by either strafing or dropping napalm bombs on the enemy. I said a remorseful goodbye to Creature and my home town and returned, reluctantly, to the painful present, smiling.

Corpsman Rector jostled me and I turned to him, smiling. He looked at me as if I had gone completely mad. Maybe I had, but what a welcome insanity it was even for the short time it lasted. I was no longer shook. I suddenly realized that it's the ability to turn off your left brain and turn on your right, just taking yourself mentally out of one unpleasant environment and putting your mind at ease in another. It's bringing back pleasant thoughts of the past, or hopes for the future that can make all the difference in combat, or any stressful situation. This sometimes is your only option for survival, the only way to save your mind, your heart and your soul.

Chapter Three

POISON PARTY

Early one beautiful summer morning I received an urgent field phone call from Army Lieutenant John Heath, a close friend of mine despite the fact he was a "dogface" army officer and I was a "jar head" marine doctor. "Dogface" or "doggie" are American terms from World War II that are used to describe soldiers in the U.S. Army. It is, they say, derived from a hang-dog or cowed expression that most army soldiers have after any of the long marches they have to walk. I am not sure where the term "jarhead" came from, most seem to think it's from the 'buzzcut' haircuts recruits have to get when they enter the marines.

John was the commanding officer of an army "8-inch" artillery battalion, which was adjacent to and in support of the marine battalion to which I was currently attached. Lt. Heath's battalion had no medical officer, so it was up to my corpsmen and me to take care of their sick and wounded. I knew that it had to be really important if John was calling me personally, someone had to be wounded or was terribly ill.

I answered the field phone expecting the worst as I waited for John's reply to my heartfelt hello.

"Hey, Doc! It's glad to hear your voice. I have a couple of sick guys on the way over and I just wanted to make sure you were there when they arrived."

"What's the matter with them, John?" I asked. I wanted to be as ready as possible for the men when they reached our battalion.

"I don't know. One of them is sort of in a coma and the other one is so dizzy he is barely able to stand. He just keeps moaning and puking." In John's voice I could hear his great concern for his men. I wanted to help them all I could, but from his description they could be sick with just about anything.

I waited and shortly after I hung up the two patients, in army fatigues, arrived on a half-track. One of the men, who was older than the other, appeared to be unconscious, his fatigues were soiled with vomitus, the smell alone was sickening. I had him carried into our medical tent on a stretcher. The other patient should have been carried in on a stretcher also, it took two men to support him as he 'walked' to where I was going to examine him. Each of the soldiers had master sergeant strips on their fatigues. It was obvious to me that my only means of finding out what could have happened was to interrogate the sergeant who was still conscious. I deeply hoped that what they had wasn't contagious. The last thing any of us needed was another enemy to fight.

"What's the matter, Sarge?" I asked as I looked into the man's bloodshot eyes. No response, he didn't hear me.

"What the hell happened to you, fella?" I questioned, almost shouting.

"I don't know, Doc," he mumbled, "My head feels funny. I can't hear so good. My ears are ringing. Everything is going round and round and I'm sick to my stomach. Damned if I'm not getting weaker by the minute." The look in his eyes slipped from fear to panic, then he retched.

What did these men have? My corpsmen started to make them as comfortable as possible while I searched my brain for what their malady could be. Then it dawned on me.

The symptoms of deafness, vertigo, and vomiting gave me a differential diagnosis limited to acute infection of the labyrinth or toxicity of the inner ear. I turned to the other sergeant lying on the cot, who I realized wasn't in a coma, as Lt. Heath had said. I opened the man's eyes and found that he had severe rotatory nystagmus, a medical term for short, jerky rhythmic movement of the eyes which occurs when the labyrinthine inner ear is irritated. His dizziness was of such a magnitude that he didn't dare move a muscle. One whiff and I knew he had been drinking. I shouted at him a few times, his hearing was nearly absent, but he did respond to the louder shouts.

Obviously they were suffering from the same malady. Both had normal temperatures. I breathed a sigh of relief, infection was very unlikely since neither had a fever and being isolated from civilization, as we all were, infectious diseases of any type were uncommon. I hadn't seen anyone with an upper respiratory infection, a cold, for at least six months. It had to be some sort of a toxic reaction, but from what? I turned again to question the younger sergeant.

"Have you guys been eating any gook food or drinking hard alcohol?"

"No, sir." The young man answered shakily, looking around at the other men in the tent.

I knew I wasn't getting anywhere with an audience of corpsmen and the usual group of curious onlookers, so I evacuated the tent of all the personnel that wasn't needed and proceeded to ask him questions.

"Come on now, Sarge. I know damned well that as sure I am standing here you've taken something to cause this. If you don't tell me what it is, how the hell am I going to treat you? This could be serious you know."

"Okay, Doc." He sighed and began to explain what had happened. "I just didn't want everyone to know about this. Me and the sergeant major were having a little party with Old Forester whiskey and water. The drinks were getting a little dry, no ice and all, so I added some wintergreen stuff, the kind you rub on sore muscles. That couldn't be what hurt us, could it?"

"Well, I don't know. Where did you get this wintergreen stuff?" I asked him.

He stared back at me as if I just started to speak another language. He wouldn't tell me. Actually, I realized, he didn't have to tell me, I was reasonably sure where it had come from. The only wintergreen flavored solution we had in the battalion was methyl salicylate. I had given Lt. John Heath a bottle of oil of wintergreen, just last week, to be rubbed on the skin for back strain.

I made sure the patients were comfortable and then called Lt. Heath on the field phone to see if his bottle was missing, it was. Having no medical books with me and not remembering the treatment and seriousness of ingesting methyl salicylate internally, I called Dr. Frick at "A" Medical

Company. After discussing it a while, we concluded that neither of us knew much about the condition other than the salicylate's affect on the labyrinth, which explained their symptoms.

As soon as I got off the phone with Dr. Frick I called and discussed the situation with Commander MacLaughlin, an internist. Commander MacLaughlin was immediately concerned.

"You had better get them down here in a hurry!" he insisted nearly yelling into the phone. "If we can't do anything for them, we'll evacuate them to the hospital ship."

I sprung into action. I didn't expect it to be that serious, but I vowed these guys would get the best care we had.

All the helicopters were busy, so my corpsmen and I loaded the two sergeants into our 'crackerbox' ambulance and we started out on what we referred to as the 'longest, dustiest ten miles in the world.' I am sure our passengers enjoyed it even less than we did.

We arrived at the 'A' Medical Company in record time. There outside was, Old Mad Mac, as he was appropriately nicknamed, pacing back and forth mumbling something about the renal complications of salicylate poisoning. A medical problem such as this was enough fuel to get Mac into one of the excited states for which he was legendary.

"What took you guys so long to get here?" he growled. "How are you feeling, doctor?" he asked. At first I didn't know what he was talking about, I had long since put my feelings, physical and mental, about my run-in with that mine to rest.

I told him I was feeling fine and started to talk about the two soldiers we just brought to him. He explained that he had intravenous fluids and a helicopter in readiness. It was his plan to evacuate the two sergeants to the 11th Army Field Hospital rather than the hospital ship, for they had a number of specialists to handle this condition and much better equipment. I agreed. Mad Mac then turn to the patients and became involved in starting the intravenous fluids and supervising the loading of the patients onto the helicopter. It was as if we no longer existed.

Feeling confident that the men were getting the best care possible and were in good hands, Corporal Wagner and I drove the ten miles back to our battalion at a much more leisurely rate of speed than our prior trip had been. When we returned to sickbay I put in a call to Lt. John Heath. As soon as I had him on the line I explained the situation;

"Say, John, your boys are in good hands. We sent them back to a 'doggie' field hospital via a whirlybird. I have no idea as to the prognosis or how long they will be hospitalized. If I were you I would put in for replacements immediately."

"Thanks a lot, Doc." He paused for a while, then continued,"Doc, I just happened to remember. I found out that an English sergeant was drinking with the other two in their little 'poison party'. I wonder how he made out?"

"Cripes, John, that sure as hell makes everything dandy, doesn't it?"

I thought a moment, we had to find the English sergeant. "Do you have any idea where this English sergeant's outfit is located? We should look into this. I am sure that his doctor won't have any idea what is ailing him since he doesn't know what he drank." There was silence on the other end of the phone.

"Well, I'm not sure, but I think they are located about two miles east of our recoil position which is about ten miles north of here," he stated with conviction. " My two men probably met this English fellow while they were setting up that position. The roads aren't that bad. I'll put Lt. Ernie Jones in charge and I'll be with you in about 15 minutes."

Lt. Heath hung up with a bang. I waited half an hour until he arrived, then John Heath, along with Corpsman HMC Taylor and I started out upon our long journey to the British unit to our northeast in our cracker-box ambulance.

The trip seemed to go on uneventfully for the first couple of miles. When we had gone about three miles and were passing in the vicinity of a foreign regiment suddenly from our right, rifle fire broke out! We listened to our first instinct and slowed down to see if it would happen again and sure enough it did. Who were these people? They were supposed to be on our side. From over head we could hear the shots flying by our ambulance from an unknown sniper out in the boonies. Most of the sniper's bullets missed, but one hit the back of the ambulance. That one bullet was enough to send Lt. Heath into orbit. His face turned a dark shade of crimson, he was very obviously bullshit. John applied the brakes so forcefully that I thought we were going to slide off the dirt road into a rice paddy.

"What the hell are you doing, John?" I yelled. "You could have gotten us killed, the sides of this road are loaded with mines, you know?"

"I know it, Doc, but these bastards have been pop-shooting at us for the past few months. This time, I'm ready for them." He grabbed his weaponry, opened the door on the driver's side and slowly dropped to the dirt road.

Lt. John Heath was certainly prepared. He had three automatic carbine rifles loaded with two 36 round clips taped together. The three carbines loaded with 72 rounds each added up to 216 shots. These clips have a slight curve. I don't know why, but I suspect it has something to do with the flow of bullets.

Lt. Heath was like a man possessed. He yelled up to us to grab rifles and join him. Chief Taylor and I, being medics, were generally not allowed to bear arms, but in this case we took exception and joined Lt. Heath on the dirt road, waiting to take aim and fire.

The lieutenant, being a combat soldier, in contrast to the Chief and I, knew exactly where the sniper fire was coming from and pointed it out to us. Without saying a word, just using hand signals, he told us to take cover at the back of the vehicle and then he crept to the front. When Chief Taylor and I had reached our cover John gave us the signal and we opened fired simultaneously. We, of course, aimed over their heads. It was after we had emptied all of our three carbines that we crept back into the ambulance and proceeded on our way. I then noticed that John had other clips in the back if we ran into any other trouble. I hoped we wouldn't.

We soon arrived at the English encampment. The camp, for the most part, was slightly on the untidy side except for this very large tent separated from the other main group of tents. We assumed that this was where we would find the commanding officer.

As we walked closer, I saw that this tent was like no other I had seen in Korea. The surrounding grounds were well-kept, planted with flowers and trees. A screened canopy-like entrance had the added protection of a screen door at each end to keep out the insects. As we reached the entrance of the tent's "front yard," a chubby, mustached major came out the door to great us. He had, to my unhidden surprise, an iced beverage in his hand.

"Come inside where it is comfortable, gentlemen," he said with a huge inviting grin on his face. HMC Taylor saluted, did an about face, stated he would be in the NCO, non commissioned officers, tent and left. Lt. Heath and I then followed the Englishman into the tent.

As we walked into the interior, the room gave us the startling, yet refreshing, sensation of being in civilization again. There was white sand on the floor and the room was screened on two sides. The furnishings consisted of easy chairs, a couch, a coffee table, bar, totem pole, a fake fireplace, and many other rustic improvisions, very effectively creating the environment of an English tavern. After the usual niceties of introduction, I told the major where we were from.

"Always good to see you Americans, you know?" the British major stated between sips of his cold drink.

"Major, do you by any chance have a sergeant who is ill?" I asked, getting straight to the point. The major couldn't hide his surprise.

"The sergeant major has been frightfully ill all day. Queer sort of thing, you know. We are waiting for a doctor." He paused and continued curiously, his voice raising slightly, "Now gentlemen, how in the world did you hear about this way over in your sector and why does it concern you?"

"Well, sir, your sergeant major and two of Lieutenant Heath's sergeants had a little party last evening. John calls it the 'poison party' and he's dead right about that. The damned fools added methyl salicylate to good whiskey. Our boys are pretty sick. We had to evacuate them by helicopter this morning," I stated and waited for his response. He said nothing so we all sat there in silence. I continued. "Would you like me to look at your sergeant?"

"By all means doctor, please." The major smiled gratefully. "It was mighty neighborly for you chaps to come all this distance. The sergeant will be more than pleased to see you, but let's have a bloody beer first. We have some in a cooler you know."

"Sure, major, I don't mind if I do." Even though I wanted to see how the sergeant was feeling, it would have been insulting if I didn't accept the drink that was offered. John and I drank our beer heartily, both of us were quite thirsty from our dusty ride. The beer was quite cool, a refreshing change, and of excellent quality. Fifteen minutes passed before I finally realized it was past time to see the sergeant.

When we got to his hut the sergeant wasn't wearing anything except a damp pair of undershorts. After the customary introductions he apologized for his lack of garb stating that the remainder of his clothing was saturated with sweat. The sergeant was a bright man and fortunately he had treated himself by forcing tremendous amounts of fluids down and now only complained of a slight ringing in his ears. He was no longer dizzy or nauseated. He was sure lucky. Before telling him all I knew I asked him what had happened.

"Sir, it's a mystery to me," he said, wiping the sweat from his brow. "I was out on a little party. Truly, I only had a few drinks, just enough to put me in the proper spirits. About 10 o'clock, I got into my jeep and started my way back to camp. I'll tell you it was a good thing I had a driver with me because if I hadn't I would be lying by the side of the road right now. Never had such a spell of dizziness and throwing up in all of my days. Frightful thing you know! Then I let loose on the other end, what a mess! I don't remember much about coming home or getting into bed, but when I woke up this morning, the dizziness and the throwing up were gone, but I was dry as the desert itself and the ringing was still in my ears. I feel much better now. The bells are beginning to leave. All I have been doing for the most part today is sweating."

I patted him on the shoulder and slowly began to explain what his "poison party" companions had done with the fixed cocktails. When I had finished I could see anger and disbelief fighting for control in his eyes. Anger finally won.

"Why those bloody bastards gave me a mickey! How do you like that now?" he expostulated. "Doc, I have one thing to ask. I, pardon the expression, puked my guts out. That's what saved me from being quite ill. Am I correct?"

I started to nod in agreement when I saw something move in my peripheral vision quite a ways away, I turned to see a short, thin man approaching in the distance. He had a pack slung over his left shoulder. As he came nearer, my attention focused on his lop ears, pointed nose and a cap several sizes too large. He stopped just a yard in front of us, clicked his heals and saluted with a snappy, palm forward, English salute.

"My name is Doctor Perkins," he stated with a grin. I was so startled by this manner of greeting that I nearly forgot to return his salute, a faux pas I wish never to bestow on a comrade in arms. After I returned his salute Dr. Perkins continued, "I presume you are Dr. Montgomery?"

I nodded in agreement.

"The Major has informed me of your presence. Right nice of you to give us a hand," he said pleasantly.

I smiled and then together we examined the sergeant. Other than an alteration in his fluid balance and the symptom of tinnitus, he seemed to be normal. The toxic reaction in his labyrinth was leaving and he had no systemic manifestations of salicylate poisoning. So, we, Dr. Perkins and I, agreed that hospitalization was unnecessary and he was going to make a full recovery.

By the time I had said goodbye to the sergeant and Dr. Perkins it was nearing 5:00 p.m. so, John and I decided to locate Chief Taylor and start on our way back to the battalion. The thought of traveling more than ten miles on that road, most of which was no more than a mile from the front line, was not my idea of a pleasant evening. I was tired and hungry. We had already missed evening chow and would be fortunate to get back before the sun went down.

After we had located Chief Taylor I offered to drive back since Lt. Heath had driven us here. We climbed into the ambulance. I geared into low four wheel drive, to ensure more comforting passage over the mud ruts in the road, and we started off. We hadn't gone more than a hundred feet when a lieutenant approached us on the run.

"I say there, Doctor, hold on for a moment!" he yelled between breaths. "The major would like to show you his appreciation over another cocktail. It won't take but a jiffy. Come on, now."

John and I discussed it and we agreed that another half an hour, more or less, at this point wouldn't make a difference. We followed the lieutenant into the officers tent and Chief Taylor left us, heading in the opposite direction calling back over his shoulder, "Give me a yell when you are ready to leave."

As soon as we walked in and my eyes adjusted to the light inside the tent I was struck again at how much like a home this place was.

The English truly knew how to exist in this, or any, "God forsaken" foreign land. I presumed this ability came from all the centuries the country had outposts of colonial rule around the globe. They certainly knew what it took to make a place have a touch of home, wherever you were. This tent was no exception. Even though I had seen it earlier that day there were still things to marvel at.

John and I sat down with the lieutenant and major and thoroughly enjoyed their conversation and cocktails of bourbon and water. So much so, that neither of us gave it a second thought when we accepted their invitation to dinner. By now it was 6 p.m. and both John and I assumed dinner was only a few minutes away. Slowly an hour passed and the novelty was wearing off for John. By this time he was giving me the old high sign in fifteen minute intervals. What was I to do, I thought angrily. I blankly ignored him for I was having a good time listening to the English accents and I was learning about their sector and manner of warfare.

Finally, at 8 p.m. on the dot, the cook entered the living area and announced dinner. We left the English tavern-like "room" and filed into the next compartment of the tent which was the dining "room". This "room," bare except for a large table, which was centrally located, covered with a linen table cloth and napkins and four place settings with real silverware and china. Just the sight of those table settings lined up in a civilized order gave me such a thrill of pleasure, part of me had almost forgotten such things existed.

The sights of color and texture, and the smells, the smells were simply heavenly. Our first course was fruit cocktail, followed by the main course, steak with mushrooms, numerous vegetables and relishes. All courses were served with an endless supply of wine, it seems every time the wine in my glass had reached the halfway mark, the 'waiter' would quickly sneak behind me and fill it up. We ended our wonderful meal with layer cake and coffee. This had been, by far, the best meal I had since leaving the States; for one thing everything hadn't all been piled onto one plate. The bubble burst when I finally looked at my watch, it was nearly 10 p.m., time to go home. Chief Taylor was sent for, and regretfully John and I said our farewells and departed the warm confines of the English tent.

As we groped in the darkness towards our jeep, the major called after us, "By the way, it's best to keep the lights off until you reach the main road."

Great, I thought sarcastically to myself, the main road was at least a half mile from here. It was dark, granted there was a full moon, but it was still too dark to maneuver a jeep correctly, especially after having a few drinks. I yelled back to the major, "How the hell am I going to see, major? The visibility is almost nil."

"I'll send Corporal Hastings along." The major replied, "He will direct you out to the main channel and head you in the right direction. Good evening, now! Come back and see us."

Soon, Corporal Hastings took his post on the hood of our vehicle and started to direct my driving. I am sure for the most part we weren't on the road fifty percent of the time. At least, I thought silently to myself, the sides of the road weren't mined. Even though Hastings and I spoke the same language, in theory that is, I was having more and more difficulty understanding him. I wasn't sure if it was the effects of the wine or what. I knew one thing though for all his bravado I was pretty certain Corp. Hastings couldn't see the road beneath us any better than we could.

Gratefully, we finally reached the main route with only a couple of additional dents in the fender, said our goodbyes to Corporal Hastings, turned on the lights and we were on our way back to camp. We were all quite happy, too happy, 'snockered' is a better word. Taylor, I gathered, had a similar drinking experience at the NCO tent, the only difference being he had gotten saturated on beer, while John and I had doused on bourbon and wine. We began singing 'Down by the Old Mill Stream' and 'I Once Knew a Sailor' for the first couple miles oblivious to the fact we were only about a half a mile from the front line. We began to hear 'incoming' up ahead and I began to think about snipers or an ambush. My happiness slowly turn to caution, so I stopped the vehicle and turned out the lights, realizing that there was enough moonlight to see by to make it back to camp. There was no way I was going to turn the lights back on.

When we finally rounded the bend which was the approach to our battalion I felt a tiring sense of relief. It was after 2 a.m. and I immediately turned on the lights so that we would be recognized and avoid getting shot by our own men.

After returning to the battalion, I picked up an extra sleeping bag for John and crawled into mine for a well welcomed sleep. We both slept through until 10 o'clock the next morning. Evidently, someone woke Chief Taylor early that morning and he had read them the riot act. He also told them to let Lt. Heath and I sleep and then grabbed a few more hours of shuteye himself. I wasn't going to tell the colonel about our little trip, but he found out about it and I had to eventually give him a full report, except, of course, the part about the "snipers".

Chapter Four

HALLOWEEN

As the soothing blanket of restful sleep slowly enveloped me I quietly remembered what tonight was, one of my favorite nights of the year, All Hallow's Eve, Halloween. The wonderful, mysterious night when ghosts and goblins walk among us under the shadow of the moon. October 31st, the night of mystery and wonder, passed me by without even a caramel apple for my trouble. No soaping of windows, no tales of the headless horsemen and creatures who go bump in the night, no trick-or-treaters banging at the front door trying to get in, not if you don't count the enemy artillery shelling us, and no candy that would last for months, nothing. Halloween in Korea had been like any other day, like any other night; no treats but, but plenty of tricks thrown at us by the enemy.

As I slowly drifted off to sleep I welcomed my dream of long ago when Halloween was filled with joy and childlike abandon, of a special night as bewitching as it was wonderful.

In West Rutland, Vermont when I was a child, on Halloween we honored the saying known only to that holiday, "trick-or-treat." If they didn't treat we, by the law of the witching hour, tricked.

In my childhood days most people in town had porches, by whatever name, piazzas, verandas, front, side or back. Whatever they were called they almost always had a roof overhead and a few wooden steps. For years, on the night devils walked the Earth, us included, we left most of the town stranded in their own homes. Every Halloween we dismantled all the porch steps we could find. It was easy to do, since dry rot was a major conspirator in our mischievous crime and it was in the spirit of the night.

We were always fast. They, the grown-ups, never caught us, but they did outsmart us. For years after our "reign of terror" most of the steps in town were replaced with marble, the most available substance in town.

Another trick that we did as children, reserved only for Halloween to give the owners a fair chance, was to sneak into a property and let their pigs loose. The pigs were just like race horses at the gate. As soon as we let them loose and they were clear of the pen they took off at full run, squealing endlessly. In our little town there were many dogs, both domesticated and strays or 'town-dogs' and all of them hated pigs. So, before long there were squealing, fat, oinking pigs being chased by a half a dozen yelping, growling, barking dogs followed closely behind by a fuming, irate, yelling pig farmer. All running like a parade down the center of Marble Street, the business section of town which coincidentally had less marble structures than Main Street, with no regards for cars, horses, or people.

Halloween was always an exciting time of year, a day I always looked forward to with a fierce anticipation. It was the one time of the year when being bad was almost the right thing to do.

Tricks were our specialty on Halloweens. We tried and did everything in the book. We played prank after prank, but only on unbelievers who had stiffed us on treats. Everything from soaping windows with hard-to-remove wax to one of my favorites, grape throwing.

Most wild and domestic purple concord grapes were ripe just about Halloween time and many Polish families in town had a grape arbor in their back yards, often with the purpose of making a bit of wine, so in the fall for us kids, getting a big bag of grapes was no problem.

Main Street ran parallel to the marble wall protecting the cemetery, leaving only the width of the marble sidewalk between the road and the marble wall. Most of us could just barely see over the wall on our tiptoes, but we waited patiently for a car to come along. When a target finally approached, off went a barrage of grapes splatting into the side of the car with a proud purple plop. Without exception the car would then screech to a halt seemingly ejecting its irate occupant who would come running after us hurling horrendous threats about the police, our parents and our grim futures if we lived that long. That was half the fun, trying to get away. They didn't stand a chance against us youngsters for we knew every tombstone in the graveyard and if need be we could zigzag through the cemetery and over the back wall up into the hills to safety.

This trick was short-lived, however, for one Halloween we had a real scare. A car drove by real slow and the barrage of grapes which were aimed at the side of the car hit the windshield instead. The driver slammed on the brakes, went out of control and knocked a telephone pole over flat with his left fender. The driver rushed out of the car in hot pursuit and we, being enthralled by the screeching brakes and crash, were a bit behind in the game. He must have been a young man for he was only steps behind us all through the cemetery. We barely made it over the wall and into the woods where he lost us.

This ended our grape throwing...for that year anyway! We did hide in the bushes on the side of the main road mostly during the summer months under the protection of the thick foliage. When a car went by, it was met by piercing police whistles, and just the same, when the car stopped, the running would start. One day in my eager exuberance I found myself blowing the whistle with all my might and its magnitude at an unsuspecting car only to slowly realize my victim was the Sheriff. He recognized me and my short life passed before me as I vainly tried to look invisible. I got off easy, though. One week of slave labor and confinement to our property.

Acres and acres of swampland with running brooks beautified the area west of our town near the marble quarries. In these swamps grow millions and maybe billions of cattails. At Halloween time, they were dry and perfect for what we referred to as a "swamp fire". If you got caught setting one of these fires it was real bad. I mean, you didn't just get hell, you had to go to court, your family was in disgrace and you were very unpopular with all the adults in town, especially the teachers. Only a few "bad" kids were involved in setting these fires. I was never involved except as a spectator, and it was a sight to remember, believe me, and we all talked about it this time of year and wondered if there would be a swamp fire.

Plans to set a swampfire had to be made very carefully and in great detail. First of all, the Sheriff and other officials in town sort of expected swampfires to be set on Halloween, so sometimes they were and sometimes they weren't. It might be the day before or the day after Halloween. It might even be a week away from this holiday.

Wind was a very important factor, for the fire had to be set so that it would travel rapidly but not towards the village. A route of entrance to and escape from the ignition site was imperative and the escape route was always directed toward one of the mountains which surrounded the town. There, from this high vantage point, the firestarters would gather with the spectators to gaze at the beautiful fire and the fire truck coming from downtown along with others from out of town.

One of our other favorite Halloween tricks for years was to tip outhouses. Back in the 1920's and early 1930's many people in our town still had outhouses and they knew on the night of Halloween they should try their best to protect them. It was common for many owners to chain a mean, spirited dog to the outhouse. This didn't stop us, of course, not when we could get our hands on ripe red meat from a barrel in the back of the butcher shop. Part of our youthful fun was getting the meat. Most of the time we would have to get it out of the barrel with a stick and a lot of coaxing and cajoling since the stench was so great it could choke a maggot. When we did complete that first task it would then take only two kids if it was a one seater, or three kids, if it was a two seater, to push over the outhouse. One boy would creep up to the dog. By the time he got close, the dog would have quit barking because he smelled the meat. He then threw the meat at the dog and ran. Then ever so slowly the other one or two boys would commando their way to the outhouse, the dog's attention being diverted from his eyes to his nose, and push the outhouse over in one quick movement. We always made sure not to push the outhouse over on the dog even if we didn't like him. We believed, even then, that all dogs were good and so-called "bad dogs" were just reflections of their masters.

Every Halloween this outhouse tipping was sort of a ritual. A ritual that ended the Halloween we got caught. The night was cold, it was dark and drizzly, and the time was right to tip some "privies". This particular outhouse was an easy target for there was no dog guarding it. So, we set about upon our evening task. We snuck up, dodging from bush to bush, applied our bodies to the selected wall and started to push. Nothing happened. Even though there were three of us pushing, nothing happened. We pushed harder, groaning against the damp wood. It started to rock, then a long groan answered us from within! We suddenly realized that there was someone in there, or something! Well, it was too late now, the occupant let out a yell and just before the outhouse took its final rock and went over, out of the door came rushing Mr. Klosiwiecz, with his pants around his ankle.

"Yaaaargh!" we screamed in unison as the dark figure came at us.

Scrambling for a foothold in the mud we took off in several directions at once as only the frightened can do. He didn't have a chance catching us with his pants around his ankles, and it was dark, so we escaped down the street. We gathered under a large chestnut tree a safe distance away, panting and sharing our version of the attack. Were we all sure it was really Mr. Klosiewicz? The enchantment of the night had started to transform our adventure, along with a good dose of boyhood adrenaline.

Halloween was a magical part of my childhood. I never let it go by since I've grown without thinking of that child I once was, how I reveled in the sheer pleasure of being alive, the magic and enjoyment I took in having fun. Gratefully and to my pure amazement that part of me, reintroduces itself to the man from time to time, and tells him the world is okay. Even in the worst of times, you can find and delight in the mystery, the magic and the miracle of life.

Chapter Five
GAMBLING

When the time in Korea became so quiet it could almost be called peaceful we played our chosen form of friendly competition, cards. My card games were limited to cribbage and I don't remember meeting a corpsman who didn't play. We never wagered for money, for there was little or none to be found, but whiskey, cigarettes, chewing tobacco, food and the like exchanged owners many times in the long days and nights. For my Marine companions, however, knowledge of cards was limited to poker, and this was a game which I only watched. My older brother once had a problem with gambling and I had this fear I might find myself running down the same path.

My brother, Dizer's (Stuart), gambling career had started honorably enough at age 12 with a friendly nickel-a-game pinball machine in Sal Glodzic's barbershop. When you won at the game, which wasn't often, the old machine would make a 'chug-chug-chug' noise and out would pour a bunch of nickels. My brother soon lived for that one symphony, that 'chug-chug-chug' noise was sweeter to him than any lyrical masterpiece from Mozart or Chopin. It was only a matter of time before the machine would clean you out, but my brother just could not see through this. He would play whenever he could get his hands on some nickels, which usually came from my father's bedroom or my piggybank. Before we knew it he was hooked and so were his friends. He was gone and his sense with him. He was treading a path we never thought he would travel, one of gambling and pilfering to play his beloved game. He soon quested, no lusted, after that one sound, for in that noise he saw hope and the promise of untold riches. After a few years the town's parents came to realize the problem and soon the machines disappeared.

Trouble had been avoided for my brother at that time but it was an ominous sign of what was to come, of what could happen if gambling took over his life and his future. Sadly it did in the next few years.

Soon after the nickel machines left town my brother and his buddies started playing cards for money. The stakes were now higher than ever for my brother, more than he ever had dreamed of playing that nickel pinball machine, just fueling the fire into a more desirable blaze. They played a game called Bid-45. I never was quite sure how they played this game and I suspect its rules and method of play have been lost over time. I sure wish I did know somebody who knows how to play it, but what I do remember about it is that it was always played anywhere there was a flat surface, even in the back seat of a car. The year my brother turned fifteen, now a three year gambling veteran, our uncle gave him a 1927 Franklin touring car which he won in a raffle for thirty-five cents. My uncle already had a Franklin, so he decided the car would go to my brother with the specific instructions that we were not to drive the car off our property until Dizer turned 16 and had his driver's license. Of course, we drove the car every chance we could get. Whenever our parents weren't around, we would tour the country, and certainly we didn't wait until he was sixteen. Soon the vehicle was dubbed 'The Flying Coffin' and stories were being told about it, legends were being formed. The back seat of 'The Flying Coffin' was large enough so that five kids could comfortably play cards on a flat piece of heavy cardboard. Since, even at the young age of 13 I realized I didn't like playing cards too much, I was most often "volunteered" to do the driving. My uncle had already taught me how to drive a hay truck, and I thought that was similar so, I did. I usually managed okay, but at times, it was pretty difficult to get the clutch engaged because I still hadn't grown too much.

Our new-found pastime soon became a difficult habit to support. Gas was twenty-five cents a gallon and twenty-five cents was often hard to come by, so we ultimately were forced into 'borrowing' any loose piece of scrap metal we could find. Often it came from the Marble Company where my father worked. We would then sell it to Mr. Metzer, the junk man, and drive to the service station to buy twenty-five cents worth of gas, one gallon. Mr. Metzer always asked us where we had gotten the scrap, but we never told him. We knew that if anyone had found out where the metal had come from my brother and I would have been in so much trouble with our father we would still be grounded to this very day.

On one of our many exploring expeditions we 'acquired' some copper wire from the Marble Company and got a very good price for it. This one act began to haunt me and I would lie awake at night, sweating goosebumps, wondering what jail was like among many other exquisite punishments.

To my dismay our father was relentless looking for the metal thieves. One evening Dad and the detective were talking in our living room about the thefts. My heart was squirming in my throat as my older brother, Dizer, and I were listening to the conversation in our pajamas from the top of the stairs. We stood there quietly, straining into every word while trying to blend into the shadows.

"Mr. Montgomery, we still don't have a lead on those metal thieves, but we think it must be some kids!" Panic! I chewed my tongue and swallowed it down again. Dizer's and my eyes locked on to each other's in frozen time.

"Well, see to it that you do find them! I want them PUNISHED!" my father demanded.

After the conversation was over and my brother and I scrambled back into our room with our hearts trailing behind us, we vowed it would end, end forever, the business of stealing metal was over! The conversation our father had with the detective had struck terror into us both, most effectively lodging into our imaginations. I always wondered if my father had planned it that way, talking just loud enough so we could easily hear, knowing somehow the culprits were under his very roof.

Since we no longer could support the car, my brother and his gambling gang (I was of no use now), tried every place imaginable to play Bid-45. They played Bid-45 on top of the woodbox. They played Bid-45 in my hen house, but the hens refused to lay in such company, so they next took over the playhouse my father was building for my sister, his one and only daughter. You can imagine how grand it was. The day it was completed Dizer moved in straight away with his gambling buddies. He did this for weeks, often forcefully evacuating my sister and her friends. She eventually complained to Dad, being completely justified, who put an end to it quickly. At the time I was surprised how she held out so long without telling. That was the end of the card playing on our property, but not the end of Bid-45.

My brother kept me abreast of their hiding places and future escapades in search of the perfect place to play. Eventually the gang moved to Mr. Pifko's pigpen (after they booted the pigs out). They discovered that if they turned over a wooden box and put a candle on it, they could deal out the hands and play very comfortably except for the smell. If you have never been in a pigpen, I must tell you, it smells like pigshit which could even make a vulture cross its eyes and go into dry heaves. It just shows what Dizer would go through to gamble. He smelled just as bad as the pigpen until midsummer when Mr. Pifko caught wind of what was going on, so to speak, and the boys were forcefully evicted. Their next haunt was the train depot. This short stay lasted less than two weeks, just the time it took the train master to find out what was going on and usher them off the property with great threats of violent bodily harm.

The boys' quest for the perfect place to play was soon over. They eventually found their haven just a few miles from our home town. They hitched a ride to a nearby lake, Lake Bomoseen, rented a row boat and played to their heart's content, as they drifted in peace, until only time itself disturbed them and sent them into their separate futures.

Chapter Six
AWOL

We had just finished a minor engagement, if you could call any fighting with the North Koreans or the Chinese minor. Whoever it was, either one or both, they were our enemies. Things had settled down some. They hadn't been rushing at us with their bugles blaring and voices screaming through the dead of night for some time. Both our side and theirs were dug in deep and except for the sporadic artillery shells slicing through the darkened sky, things were quite peaceful.

At the time we had a Janesway Hut set up for the treatment of minor wounds and triage patients who would eventually be referred back to the MASH units either by helicopter or field ambulance. The Janesway Hut used in combat is indispensable and a God-send. The hut is essentially a quonset hut-type tent which has insulated fabric 'walls', wooden floors, and is very comfortable both in warm weather and in cold. Three corpsmen worked with me in the Janesway hut, and for the most part, we kept these tents below the battalion level in the vicinity of the regiment and closer to the action.

One particular sunny day, everything was shipshape in the sickbay, so we decided to try our luck at fishing to pass the time. We had already found our source of fishing line, a couple of spools of white thread, and scrounged up some suitable poles, but no hooks. We thought about it collectively. There was a very good supply of surgical needles, which could easily be turned into fishing hooks with a little help from a needle holder, which is like pliers, to bend the hooks in just the right place. It worked. There was one draw back, though. They had no barbs, so it would be hard to keep one's fish on the hook once we caught him, but beggars can't be choosers. We decided for bait we would use canned ham and some grub-like creatures from under some rocks. We were ready. I felt just like a little kid again.

We were headed for the Imjin River, the sky was the perfect shade of blue and our spirits were high. The four of us, Beauchamp, Rector, Caps and I, walked single file in a path made between the rice paddies. None of us even thought of straying from the path. All of us had seen the damage a land mine could do if you stepped on one, and the rice paddies were, more often than not, infested with them. We were well-armed both with our fishing poles and fire arms, 45 automatic pistols and carbine rifles with 36 round clips.

We soon approached the Imjin river and our single file line spread out into walking side by side. At this point the river seemed to be about thirty-five yards wide. There were times a while back that some of the corpsmen and marines would come to the river, strip and go for a swim. This went on for a while until one day a group of Marine PFC's were all killed by enemy snipers. I don't know why we thought we were safe fishing at the same point, maybe since we would have our clothes on and rifles out and handy.

We settled down on the bank, placed our trusty carbines at our sides and started to fish. We basked in the morning sun as time slowly crept by, our conversations quiet, our thoughts occasionally wandering. Somewhere my mind slowed down, actually I was nearly asleep when all of a sudden I heard a yell thinly disguised in a whisper. It was Caps.

"Shit! Everyone keep down!"

Instinctively we grabbed for our rifles and flatten to the earth, our chests molding to the damp, cool ground.

I whispered back to Caps, "What's going on?"

His answer was one word, but it spoke volumes, "Gook!"

We quietly snapped a round into the chamber of our guns and slowly pushed the safety off with the index finger of our right hands. We waited in silence... waiting for something, anything to happen. Caps broke the tension-filled stillness with a nerve grating whisper.

"There's a friggin' gook helmet down there about 40 yards and it is moving this way."

I peeked and sure enough there was a shiny helmet bobbing along as the person walked straight toward us. My hand grabbed my rifle tighter to my body, my trigger finger moved into position and my eyes searched the enemy for any signs of aggression. My mind raced, asking questions no one could answer right now. Has he seen us? Did he have a grenade? If so how many? Did he have comrades close by? Were we going to have to shoot him? Who would do it? We could take him prisoner, right?

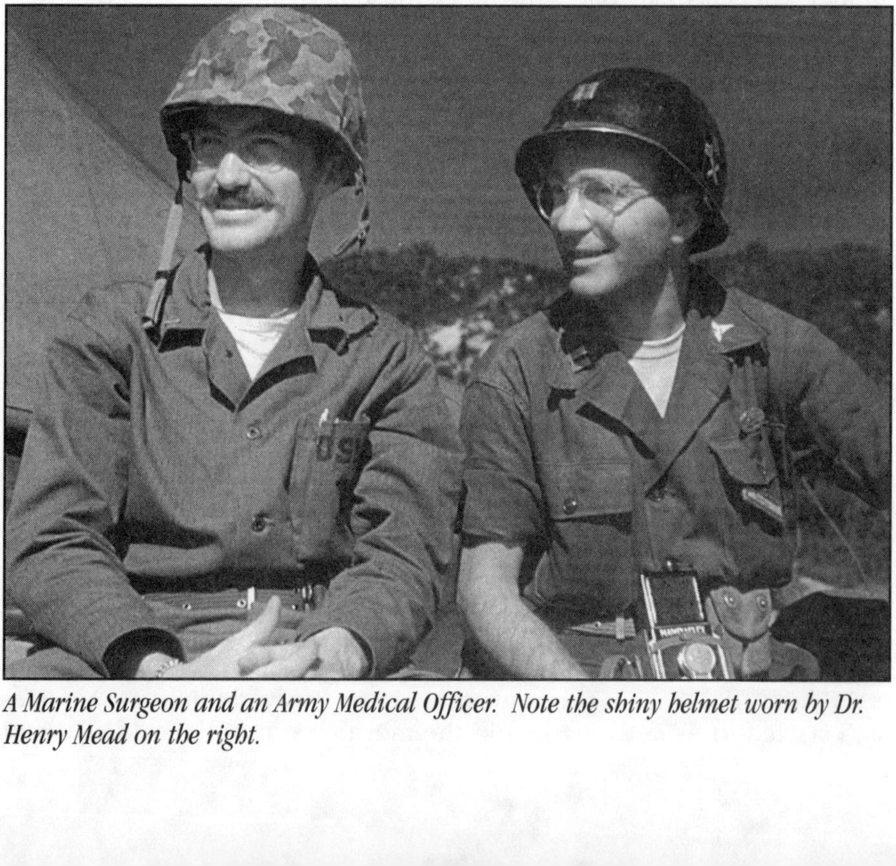

A Marine Surgeon and an Army Medical Officer. Note the shiny helmet worn by Dr. Henry Mead on the right.

That was pretty hard to do even if you were trained for it, and none of us were. I decided not to shoot until absolutely necessary and gave an order not to fire until we could see clearly what we were shooting at. The men bristled slightly, I am sure the seasoned corpsmen with me didn't like taking orders from an officer who was really a doctor.

The man in the helmet was walking along as if he hadn't a care in the world or as if he didn't care who in the world shot him. We waited until he was about 25 yards away, then Caps, standing it no longer, yelled, "Who's there and what the f— do you want?"

The helmeted man stopped dead in his tracks. Then a friendly, and more surprising, an American voice answered, "I am Captain Mead. I am looking for a marine doctor!"

The men all looked at me and I took a step out from behind my hiding place and yelled back at him over the yards of distance.

"Are you looking for just any marine doctor or someone in particular?"

"I am looking for Dr. Montgomery," he yelled back hopefully. "Do any of you know him?"

I was dumbfounded. This man was walking in the middle of a war zone looking for me. I started to walk closer, that is when I recognized him. It was Henry "Hank" Mead in an army uniform, unarmed except for a pistol. He had been my closest friend throughout medical school.

"Well, Hank, you found him," I answered as I lifted my camouflaged helmet off my head grinning from ear to ear. Recognition, then relief spread across his face and we ran toward each other and embraced like the old friends that we were. We then stepped back and took a look at each other.

"What the hell are you doing here in jarhead country?" I asked jokingly.

"It's a very long story, Bill," Hank remarked wearily. I nodded and took him over to meet the rest of my party, not wanting to push for any answers until he was ready. Beauchamp, Rector and Caps went back to the river and started to fish again as Hank and I sat a ways back and he began to tell me his story.

"I got a "Dear John" letter from Sally and went apeshit, I took one of my medic's, a weapons carrier truck and drove sixty miles across the front looking for you. I had to talk to someone who knew me, who knew Sally. Someone I trusted." Hank then paused as if trying desperately to find the words to continue. "Before leaving I had our communications officer call your division headquarters to find out your location. Then I just started out in this direction. I don't believe I found you."

I couldn't find the words to console him. I just smiled briefly and we sat there in silence for a while, letting him know he could talk to me all he wanted.

At medical school we were divided into groups of four for human anatomy study, each group having one cadaver. Hank and I were in the same group and thus got to know each other like brothers that first year.

It was during our junior year that Hank met Sally, a college student from a nearby school. They fell in love virtually right away. They were married our senior year and moved to a small city in Rhode Island after our internship, where he set up general practice about the same time I started general practice in Vermont. We had both become very busy with our lives and had lost touch in the past two years, only hearing from each other on holidays and birthdays.

I had heard that Hank had been called into service about the same time I was and after a fairly adequate training in the army was sent to the front line in Korea.

Hank slowly began to relate the story of what had happened to him, what led up to him being absent without leave and why he had searched around Korea for me. He told me that he was beginning to cope with the dead and wounded and what seemed sometimes like endless work. He said the only thing that had kept him going was the thought he would be back with his wife when all this was over, then the letter came. He said it had hit him like a freight train. The thing was he didn't see it coming. There were signs, but he just didn't read them. He had been getting letters from his wife on a regular basis the first year he was stationed in Korea, then slowly the intervals between each correspondence became longer. He thought she had just gotten busy or the mail was slow, then the "Dear John" letter arrived. Evidently, she had been having an affair with another man in town during Hank's absence and had fallen in love with him. She wrote Hank in the letter that she was going to leave him and get a divorce so she could marry this man. I watched Hank as he told me this heart wrenching story of love, loss and betrayal, I couldn't imagine what kind of person could be as cruel as this....to send such a letter to a man in combat. Half-heartedly I thought, "maybe that is where the expression 'all is fair in love and war' began." One thing I did know - both stink, when it turns out like this.

I had to help Hank out of this one. I went back to my corpsmen, picked up my carbine rifle and told them that I was going back to see the colonel about Hank and they could stay and fish if they wanted to. They didn't. They had overheard some of our conversation, so they knew what was going on and decided to come back to camp with us.

Hank was a mess by the time he and I reached Colonel Honzowitz's tent. The extent of what he had done by going AWOL was starting to hit him. Colonel Honzowitz was in his tent working on his maps, he was a brilliant Marine and almost invariably several steps ahead of the enemy. My request to enter his tent was granted and I introduced Hank. I began to explain to the colonel, who knew me quite well, and could tell by the expression on my face that I indeed had a serious problem. He stood up, shook hands with both Hank and me, and told us to have a seat as he mixed us each a martini. Hank began to visibly relax and was quite impressed that the colonel would fix us a drink and a martini at that. Little did he know that Colonel Honzowitz somehow always had, for his guest, a straight up martini with an olive. I began to tell the colonel Hank's story as he handed us our drinks. I made an impassioned plea on Hank's behalf, telling Colonel Honzowitz about our long friendship and the reason why he had gone AWOL. I finished and waited for the colonel to answer. Hank had stopped drinking and was holding his breath.

The Colonel studied us for a second, and then said, "Well let's see now. What can we do about this? This doesn't seem to be too bad of a problem....let me get on the horn and see if I can find your colonel." Colonel Honzowitz asked Hank for the name of his commanding officer and his exact location. Hank let the answer fly out with the breath he had been holding. I let out a deep sigh realizing just then I had been holding my breath, too.

Colonel Honzowitz contacted our communications sergeant on the phone and told him to call Marine Division headquarters and have him transfer to Army headquarters. It wasn't fifteen minutes before the colonel was talking to Hank's commanding officer. He and the colonel seemed to hit it off quite well. I note that they avoided any conversation concerned with their locations or activity. Finally Colonel Honzowitz said, "Okay, I owe you one." and hung up.

He turned to us and explained that Hank was now on leave for three days and that there were no charges against him. Hank smiled broadly, he seemed to get younger by ten years before my very eyes, he was back to his young self. The colonel then said, "You gentlemen have any booze?"

"Yes, Sir, a little," I replied not knowing exactly what his question meant.

"Well then men," he said smiling, "Take this bottle of Scotch and go have a party."

"Thank you sir, thank you," I said gratefully as I shook his hand, took the Scotch, and went out the door with my good friend to try to forget about the war.

Chapter Seven

GENERAL PRACTICE

Hospital Corpsmen Beauchamp, Rector and I were sitting in a Janesway Hut one hot day near the 38th Parallel in Western Korea with not much to do. They were both bright, young men and not yet 21 years of age. I am sure both were thinking about taking advantage of their interest in medicine and the GI bill to enter college when and if they returned to the United States. They wanted to be doctors.

"Say, Doc," Rector asked, "What's it like going to medical school and being in general practice like you were before you came to Korea?"

"Rector, the first year of medical school is a bitch," I explained, "or at least it was for my class. Anyone who did not study seven days a week, or had a girlfriend didn't make it. When we started there were forty in the class, at the end of the first year, there were thirty-three. The second and third year were a little bit more clinically oriented. By the end of the fourth year, most of us felt and acted like doctors. There is no way to describe internship. Sleep only every other night and often did 56 hours of straight work on the weekend. It is impossible to describe an internship," I repeated emphatically as I continued trying, "You don't think you are going to live through it, but you do.

"After completing my internship and taking a miniresidency in obstetrics, gynecology, general surgery and neurosurgery, I returned to my hometown, West Rutland, Vermont, for a try at general practice."

Not used to talking much about myself, I stopped and scrutinized Beauchamp's and Rector's faces carefully to ascertain whether or not I should continue with what could be a rather lengthy story. Beauchamp

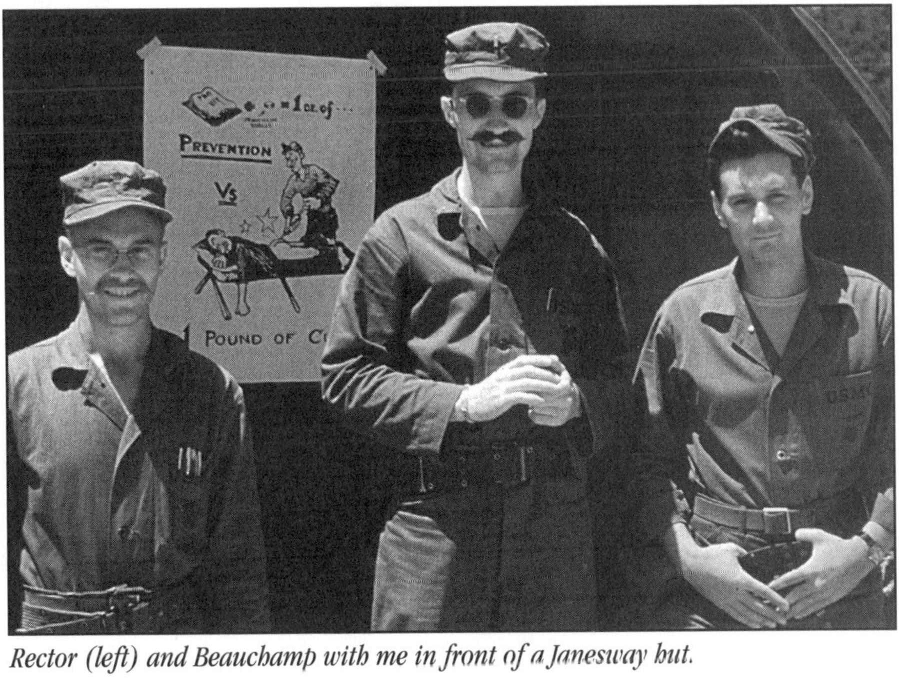

Rector (left) and Beauchamp with me in front of a Janesway hut.

was chomping his gum at a frantic pace eager to jump into every word. Rector lay back twirling a toothpick around his tongue, looking quite content and soaking it all up.

I decided to continue. I was certain that I eventually wanted to become a surgical specialist, but couldn't decide on the specialty. I was not quite 25 years old and there is no question that I probably looked a lot younger. Dr. Carol B. Ross was 85 years old then, and had been in practice in this small town for more than 65 years. He was almost completely deaf, but could read without glasses. He gladly gave up his practice so that he could enjoy fishing and his favorite hobby, reading Wild West magazines. Dr. Ross's office consisted of an isolated one story building which was about 20 x 30 feet. The building was wired for electricity, but had no running water or toilet. We started by digging a cesspool which was made of white marble, as was most everything else in town, sidewalks, foundations, library, school and churches. I put in running water and had the building made over into a waiting room, examining room and consultation room where I placed my newly purchased encyclopedia of medicine, surgery and specialties plus all of my textbooks from medical school. I don't believe there was ever a day that I did not refer to those books. I was a neophyte and knew it.

"Very few patients crossed my threshold the first week. The second week, in the middle of my afternoon office hours, I was sitting at my desk considering growing a mustache so I would look older, when two relatives brought in a lady by the name of Eva Capron, who was dying from tuberculosis. They carried her directly into my examining room and placed her on the table. During my training I had seen a number of cases of pulmonary tuberculosis. Eva's lungs, however, were not the problem. She had multiple draining sinuses at the belt level which drained a green foul-smelling discharge. Why they hadn't called and asked me to make a house call was not clear. She had been taken care of by a general surgeon in a nearby community. His treatment consisted of repeated blood transfusions in order to keep her alive.

"Streptomycin had just come out a few years earlier and was being used in tuberculosis sanatoriums as therapy for pulmonary tuberculosis. I consulted my encyclopedia and medical school textbooks and there was no information concerning this drug. The town's drugstore was directly across the street from my office."

I gave the druggist a call, 'Victor, do you have any streptomycin? Great! Would you mind getting the literature out on it so that I can do a little fast reading?' Victor and I had not been too far apart in the West Rutland school system and had become great friends after I returned to begin general practice. I spent much of my spare time with him either in my office or in his store. He had one vial of streptomycin and the literature that came along with it and could get me more in one day. One gram of streptomycin administered intramuscularly each day seemed to be the correct dose. The family insisted on bringing Eva to my office for these daily injections for the first two and a half weeks. Thereafter she became so dizzy that I had to make housecalls to administer the streptomycin. After 26 consecutive days of treatment, the sinuses stopped draining and began to heal. Six weeks later, Eva's dizziness improved sufficiently so that she could be up and around and her draining sinuses had closed and healed over completely.

"Now, there's one thing I forgot to tell you about Eva Capron. She was the town gossip. Instant success! I had it made! Eva's telephone was busier than ever and within a few weeks my practice increased from a few patients to a full office. It was necessary for me to extend my evening office hours from 8 to 10 o'clock in the evening.

"Two years later, in August, which was towards the end of my general practice days, I decided to take a day off on my birthday. I drove to Lake Bomoseen, rented a boat, and spent the day fishing. The fishing wasn't too good, but the sun was warm and it was a real relaxing day, great to get away from the constant strain and stress of practice, until 2 p.m. At this time, I saw a single enginepontoon airplane coming up the lake toward me at full speed for a takeoff. They lifted off the water and turned sharply to the right, then proceeded to crash into the woods directly across the lake. Evidently, there was water in their right pontoon. I rowed back to my car and drove around the lake to find a crowd of people. We all hiked up into the woods to find two very seriously injured men. Someone had already called for an ambulance. We administered first aid and fortunately I had my medical bag in the car so I could relieve their pain and give first aid to their wounds. It must have been 4:30 p.m. before they were in the ambulance and we were on the way to the hospital which was approximately 8 miles away. A general surgeon took over their care and I assisted him in the operating room.

"It was 10 o'clock when I reached home. I had no fish and I was tired. There was a message for me to call Eva Capron. I telephoned to learn that Eva had fallen in the morning and they thought most likely that she had fractured her upper arm. She wouldn't let anyone care for her, informing them that it was my birthday and she would wait until I returned from fishing. An X-ray taken at the hospital showed a fracture of her humerus. The treatment for this fracture was a hanging arm cast. I took the cast off six weeks later and Eva was as good as ever. The fracture, by the way, was on her left arm so it didn't interfere with her telephone activities whatsoever. I later learned that the two men injured in the airplane crash recovered, but I suspect they both had some degree of disability."

Then I told Beauchamp and Rector more general practice stories, "Every small town, such as West Rutland, has at least one town drunk. One such gentleman, whose first name was Joe, and not too much older than I, would often wander in just as I finished office hours at 9:30 or 10:00, or later in the evening. I usually managed to get him out of the office and close up within fifteen minutes so it was never any real problem. Also I saw this as a challenge to get him off the bottle, for he was potentially a very productive member of the community.

"It seems one night I got a call about 10 p.m. in the evening from Katherine Cane who said she was bleeding from her mouth rather profusely. Katherine Cane's nickname was "Pooper". How she got this name is a mystery to me but everyone called her Pooper behind her back. She was my eighth grade school teacher. Needless to say, with her personality, she was a sitting duck for practical jokers and we played many of them on her during my year in the eighth grade. I was quite honored that she would call me to care for her since there was another doctor in town, who by the way, took an immediate dislike to me after he saw that my waiting room was filled most evenings and especially after the head Polish priest called me one night for an illness."

"What happened, Katherine?"

"I don't know, William. I woke up with a start, coughed, and realized that I was bleeding from my mouth."

"I think we had better go to the hospital, Katherine," I said plainly.

"No! Please," she pleaded, "let's go to your office first. Maybe you can stop it there."

"I went to Ms. Cane's house and she was indeed bleeding profusely from her mouth. I placed her in my car with a towel over her face and drove her to the office. I had in the office a suction machine, a hyphercator, which is a cautery machine, and a flashlight. When I looked in her throat with a flashlight and the suction, I could see that she was bleeding from a rather large varicose dilated vein in the back of her throat. I attempted to stop this bleeding, but was unsuccessful for it was impossible to use the flashlight, the suction and the cautery at the same time with only two hands. I even tried it with the flashlight in my mouth! I heard a rumble out in the waiting room and opened the door to see my friend Joe who was only moderately intoxicated.

"Joe, come on in! I need your help," I told him. "Now you just take this flashlight and shine it into Katherine's throat so I can see what I'm doing." Joe held the flashlight, managing to illuminate the pharynx about 50% of the time, but this allowed me to suction out the blood and then cauterize the vein and stop her bleeding. Katherine then proceeded to vomit up the blood in her stomach which was a good thing.

"Joe, thanks a lot," I said, "I couldn't have done it without you."

"That's OK, Doc, anytime," Joe grinned.

I could tell Joe was real proud of himself. Katherine didn't look too anemic so I brought her home and that was the end of the incident.

The next day I learned to use a head mirror. I had been instructed to do so during my exposure with Dr. McMann, who was chief of Ear, Nose and Throat Surgery at the University of Vermont Medical School, but like most general doctors, abandoned its use. I learned that the head mirror was a wonderful instrument. You could use the light from a lamp or light bulb or even a flashlight if you instructed someone to hold it properly. This frees up both hands for work.

"Joe, by the way, did sober up about a year later and became the town tax collector. The last time I saw Joe was approximately 10 years ago. I went back to my hometown for a visit and decided to go down to Sal Murtie's for a haircut. Joe was sitting there with his hat on as usual, and greeted me as did everyone else in the barber shop. After Sal had finished with my haircut, Joe asked me if I noticed anything different about him. I said I thought he looked pretty well. He then turned his head and showed me that he had no left ear. Evidently he had a cancer on his ear and someone had chopped it off, which I suspect is good treatment.

"Doc," he asked, "aren't you supposed to be an ear specialist?" He had me.

I often wonder whether or not Beauchamp or Rector ever went to medical school. Certainly they had the smarts and personality to do so, but did they have the drive and persistence it takes to become a doctor? Most likely I will never know.

Chapter Eight
JANIC SMOLINSKI

I next told Beauchamp and Rector about the day Janic (pronounced Yonik - John in English) Smolinski was hit in the head with a derrick hook. The call came at exactly 4:35 in the afternoon from the quarry. I was examining a patient and there were more out in the waiting room. I looked up at the clock when the phone rang. On the other end of the phone was a very excited Vermont Marble Company quarry worker, "Doc! There's been an accident down in the main quarry and I think you should come right away!" He hung up.

The people in the waiting room had also heard the phone ring and when they saw the look on my face they knew that there was no way they were going to get to see me that afternoon. Country people are really great. They have a compassion for their fellow human beings which I quite often fail to see in the city where I am living now. I didn't have to say anything.

They stood up and prepared to leave even before I got to say, "There's an emergency in the main quarry."

I was not surprised when someone asked, "What happened, Doc? Is it bad? Who's hurt? How many?" They cared.

"Folks, I don't know but I am sure you will find out shortly after I do. Come back this evening - no, maybe you'd better call first to find out whether I am here or still in the hospital... better still, come on back tomorrow."

I ran out to my 1947 Plymouth. My siren (courtesy of the state police) cleared the road for me as I sped to the main quarry which was only two miles west of the town on the way to Whipple Hollow.

Three quarry workers were waiting for me at the edge of the quarry. I grabbed my medical bag and joined them.

In order for me to explain the next sequence, it is necessary for me to describe this main quarry. It is the largest quarry in the world. The opening on the surface is 150 feet square and it goes down to a depth of 300 feet, then expands laterally for a square mile at the bottom. To prevent a collapse of any portion, the bottom is divided into large rooms, each about the size of a football field. The partitions separating these marble rooms are ten feet thick and have an opening in the center through which are laid railroad tracks. The railroad tracks serve to move the marble from where it is quarried to the center of the quarry. Here it can be lifted from the heavy-duty railroad flatbed car by the derrick, up 300 feet and out of the quarry. The derrick is much like the ones you see being used with the construction of large buildings today. The cable is made of very heavy twisted steel. On the end of the cable is a steel hook weighing about 50 pounds.

There are two ways to descend to the bottom of the quarry. One is by way of wooden steps which zigzag down one side of the quarry wall. This is a very long walk down and a much longer walk back up. The second way to descend is on the end of the derrick cable. A seven foot square steel platform has a steel loop welded to each corner. Four equal length pieces of chain are attached to each corner loop and then to a large heavy loop above. This heavy loop is attached to the derrick hook making for a nice vehicle which can carry six to eight men. I stepped onto the platform which was on the ground at the edge of the quarry along with the three workers.

The first ride down to the bottom of the quarry on this platform is scary, or maybe I should say frightening. All is well when you step onto the platform when it is still on the ground at the edge of the quarry. Then you start to rise and the platform sways back and forth as you clear the metal fence around the edge of the quarry. This swing increases as the platform reaches the center of the quarry. It feels a little bit like a ride on the end of a clock pendulum. The first advice to a neophyte is 'Don't look down! Look at me and keep talking!' When I was in high school I worked down in this very same quarry one summer. Being the nut that I am I looked down on my first descent and want to tell you I wanted "out". What if the derrick clutch malfunctioned, or a chain slipped or broke? A 300 foot fall. Anyway, by this time I was an old hand and rather enjoyed a ride on this platform.

"What happened down there, Jake?"

"Janic Smolinski got hit on the head by the swinging derrick hook. It knocked him clean off his feet and he hasn't moved a muscle since. He is unconscious."

"Are you sure he isn't dead?"

"No, he is breathing a bit. Lot's of bleeding, though."

I looked up at the hook and could see no blood or hair. Big John Smolinski was too old to be working down here. He must have been well over 60 years of age. Obviously he didn't see the hook coming, but on the other hand, neither did anyone else. My thoughts went back to the summer after my senior year in high school when I was working in another marble quarry and a similar accident occurred. This was a new quarry which I had helped with at its inception. I can remember that summer like it was yesterday. First, we cut down the trees with chain saws, then the dozer came in and cleared the dirt off the marble surface. Following this I was introduced to a jack hammer and made holes in the surface marble approximate 6 feet deep. These were packed with dynamite, a dynamite cap packed into the top of each and then the hole was plugged with a piece of tapered wood. All the wires were connected and run 150 feet away where they joined an ignition apparatus situated behind a large tree. Most of the time, because I was a kid and possibly because I was the son of the boss, they let me push the plunger to set off the dynamite. I had been instructed not to return to the dynamite site for at least ten minutes after the blast for the fumes were rather irritating. I forgot one day and returned a few minutes after the blast. They were right. I threw up for half an hour.

The dynamite broke up the surface marble into large chunks. These had to be broken up into smaller pieces with a ten pound sledge hammer, and I want to tell you, this is a real art. You have to find the grain of the marble, and just keep hitting along this grain, and all at once the marble will split.

That summer I learned much from the Polish quarry workers. From time to time the foremen and sometimes my father would come by to check on progress. Years later I learned that they had a little joke about me. "It's hard to tell whether Bill is swinging the sledge hammer or if the sledge hammer is swinging Bill!" At this point I was almost 6 feet tall and weighed less than 130 pounds.

Getting back to a similar accident which occurred in this new quarry, I was facing the edge of the quarry, fairly close to the wall, rolling a Bull Durham cigarette. No one was accepted as one of the gang in the quarry in those days if you couldn't roll a Bull Durham cigarette with one hand. Some of you may remember Bull Durham. It was fairly good tobacco which came in a small cloth pouch with a purse string on the top. To one end of the purse string was attached a paper tag with a picture of a bull on it. The tobacco pouch was housed in your shirt pocket while the string and the tag with the bull hung outside. I was looking the other way while the hook was down in the quarry to bring up a piece of marble. The hook was swinging in a broad pendulum. Jim Zolostoski was not looking either and the hook hit him square on the side of the head. Observers say he staggered, stood up straight, and then went over like a Bugs Bunny cartoon, flat on the ground. He was dead.

Back in the main quarry where we were descending very rapidly, so much so that it almost took my breath away, just before hitting the bottom, the derrick operator put on the brake slowly and we eased to the floor of the quarry. He was good.

There was John. Someone had put their coat over him and another coat was serving as a pillow. The latter was quite bloodsoaked. John was not moving, nor did he respond to my words or physical stimulation. There was a large gash in his right temporal region. I examined his eyes and the right pupil was dilated, the left was normal and reacted properly to light stimulation. His breathing was very shallow, almost imperceptible. "Is he dead, Doc?"

"No, but let's get him topside in a hurry. Did any of you call an ambulance?"

"Yes, it should be here by now."

Four men carefully lifted John onto the platform. No one was working. They all stood around watching every move I made. There must be something fascinating about a doctor. These men, most of whom I had worked with when I was a teenager, were no longer my buddies. I was now a doctor. Janic had been there, too. The M.D. degree was some sort of a barrier between us which I never fully understood. I can still picture these men standing around with their white faces, not from fear or faint, but because they were covered with white marble dust. There were a few linear streaks on some of their faces below their eyes which had been made by tears. They loved Janic.

I can remember being covered from head to foot with this dust when I was working in this same quarry. Marble dust, in contrast to granite dust (which can cause lung disease), is not irritating or dangerous to your health. My father always told me it built strong bones because of the calcium. Marble is calcium carbonate.

My best memories of working in the marble quarry, other than my association with these fine people, was coming up on the platform in the late afternoon after a hard day's work with other workers. As I mentioned previously, the platform could accommodate up to eight workers and occasionally ten. All were in a jovial mood. Some had chunks of ice on their backs to be used in their ice chests at home. Down at the bottom of the quarry, the temperature is always exactly 27 degrees fahrenheit and ice was readily available.

Once on top, we all raced for the air hose which was twice the diameter of a garden hose and connected to an air compressor. The first worker to get there would hose off the next, beginning with his hair and working down to his boots. It was his turn next. All this made for a big cloud of white dust.

We loaded Janic into the ambulance and soon were on our way to the Proctor Hospital six miles distant. John was still not moving, but he had a fair pulse and was still breathing. I inserted a needle into an arm vein and connected this to tubing which led to a bottle of normal saline solution.

Once at the hospital, the nurses and I wheeled him directly to the X-ray department. There were no orderlies in those days. The nurses did everything. The two marble workers who were with us wanted to come in with me, but were instructed by Florida La Frances, the head nurse, to stay in the waiting room. Both, by the way, were still covered with marble dust.

Florida took a skull series and then developed the film. A plain skull series is somewhat difficult to interpret. Today a CAT scan and/or an MRI would show exactly what was going on inside the skull. We didn't even have polytomes in those days, which is an X-ray machine made known to much of the public by its usage in a movie entitled, The Exorcist. The front view X-rays showed a definite shift of structures to the side opposite his injury. The side view showed a couple of fracture lines on the side of the injury.

We needed a neurosurgeon. I picked up the phone and told the operator who I was and asked that she locate for me a Dr. Les Wallman in Burlington, Vermont. Dr. Les Wallman was one of the professors of neurosurgery at the medical school and had been my instructor.

Soon, he came on the phone, "Hey, Les! I have a rather severe head injury and I think there is a subdural hematoma, (a collection of blood under the brain covering), but I am not certain. I don't think he could take the 66 mile ride to Burlington." Les must have been in rare form, for neurosurgeons as a rule, do not like to operate away from their own environment. He said he would be right down.

Les was there in less than 90 minutes with all his equipment. He looked at the X-ray and agreed with my diagnosis. I called Dr. Fergosi, who was a general practitioner with a lot of experience in anesthesia. I shaved John's head and cleaned the wound with antiseptic while Les arranged his equipment, discussing it with Florida La Frances, who was also the operating room circulating nurse. Florida put his instruments in the sterilizer while Les and I scrubbed, then prepared and draped John for surgery. There was no need for Dr. Fergosi to give any anesthesia at the beginning of the operation for John was still unconscious.

It was good to see Les. While we were scrubbing in preparation for surgery and during intervals we talked about some of the cases we had together when I was training with him.

I injected local anesthesia into the skin around the laceration and the region in the scalp which would be incised to form a flap which in turn would expose the skull. Les asked me to make the incision and elevate the flap. Once the self-retaining retractors were in place and the skull exposed, we made four holes, 3/4 inches in diameter in the skull with an ingenious drill bit which cuts a hole through the bone of the skull and then stops. It does not enter the underlying soft tissue which is called the dura or brain covering. The bit stock is exactly the same as that used by a carpenter except it is all metal so that it can be sterilized. Today we have electric drills.

The next step was to tunnel under the skull between all four holes. Then a special wire saw is passed with a guide to protect the dura between two of the holes. The two ends of the thin wire saw (Gigli saw) have a loop which is attached to a handle. By pulling from one end and then the other, this saw cuts through bone like a knife through butter. Woodsmen often carry this type of saw in their knapsack to cut small trees. Les took over after the four saw cuts had been completed and removed the bone to expose a window of dura. He incised the dura and began removing a large clot of blood, then started the tedious task of identifying and stopping the bleeders. This took hours. Neurosurgeons are notoriously slow workers. I know because I have operated with them most of my life. Slow but sure is the name of the game. Neurosurgery cannot be hurried.

At the end of the operation the dura was sutured together and the piece of bone replaced. We put in the last skin stitch just before 2 a.m. Florida had coffee and cookies waiting for us. I tried to get Les to stay in the hospital or come home with me. He insisted on driving back to Burlington.

John came to on the first postoperative day and left the hospital in two weeks. He was, however, never the same. I made frequent house calls to check on him for six months after his injury. Dilantin had to be prescribed to prevent seizures. He was able to work in his garden and around the house a bit. The company gave him a full wage the rest of his life. He lived many years and enjoyed being with his family and they were thankful to have him home and alive.

Chapter Nine
"MAE WEST"

The hours that had just passed seemed to blend together in my mind. The tasks which I had been performing for the past several hours, though important to each of my patient's health, had become endlessly monotonous. I was in the middle of cleaning and repairing a rather large wound on a marine's thigh when my mind threatened mutiny. I had to stay fairly focused, I told myself, but I knew that if I had to I could have done this procedure blindfolded. A conversation was out of the question for the corpsman who was assisting me and the other doctor who was giving the anesthesia were was as tired as I was, and had lost the ability to talk lucidly long ago. The blood vessels in the patient's thigh had been ligated and the cutting part of the operation completed. All that remained was to bring the edges of the skin together. We had orders from the division surgeon that all wounds were to be roughly approximated (closed) and we were to use stainless steel suture material. The task was tedious at best and required very little left brain function. I finally gave in and let my mind wander back to a time when I had done this procedure for one of the first times, back to my days as a general practitioner when I had a patient nicknamed, "Mae West."

Mae was tall (5'8") and overweight. Actually, some referred to her as being fat, but certainly, she was not the saggy, baggy, pot-bellied type of fat, for her excess adipose was distributed in all the right places, accentuating her natural curves and valleys to perfection. The result was a very sensuous woman. To top it off, she moved around like a sleek young lioness. When she walked by, all the correct parts moved in synchrony (especially her rear end) with a grace that made her easy to look at, and an educated style with a certain "something" that begged all to take notice.

Mae was the daughter of a very conservative Polish family who handled her with a tight rein. She had numerous suitors all of whom had been rejected, not by her but by her father. She remained unmarried until she was twenty-six years old when finally her father lost his tight rein over his daughter. She ran off and married a "know nothing" named Seth, who was no taller than 5'4". She was happy, at least to get out from under her father's thumb.

Seth and Mae settled on a farm in Chippenhook on the outskirts of town and made their living selling eggs, milk, butter and the like. Their vegetable garden rendered them a handsome profit during the summer.

It was said that one of Mae's favorite possessions was a bull who weighed well over 1200 pounds with beautiful horns as well as some other most prized ornaments that are attached to a prized bull.

Mae, for some reason, never allowed her husband to walk with her. She made him walk more than six feet behind her, and he obeyed. This was against all traditions I knew of, but she always led the way, and Seth didn't seem to mind too much for he had one of the best views in town. At least that's how we all had it figured out.

One bright summer day Mae and Seth and the bull set out on their way

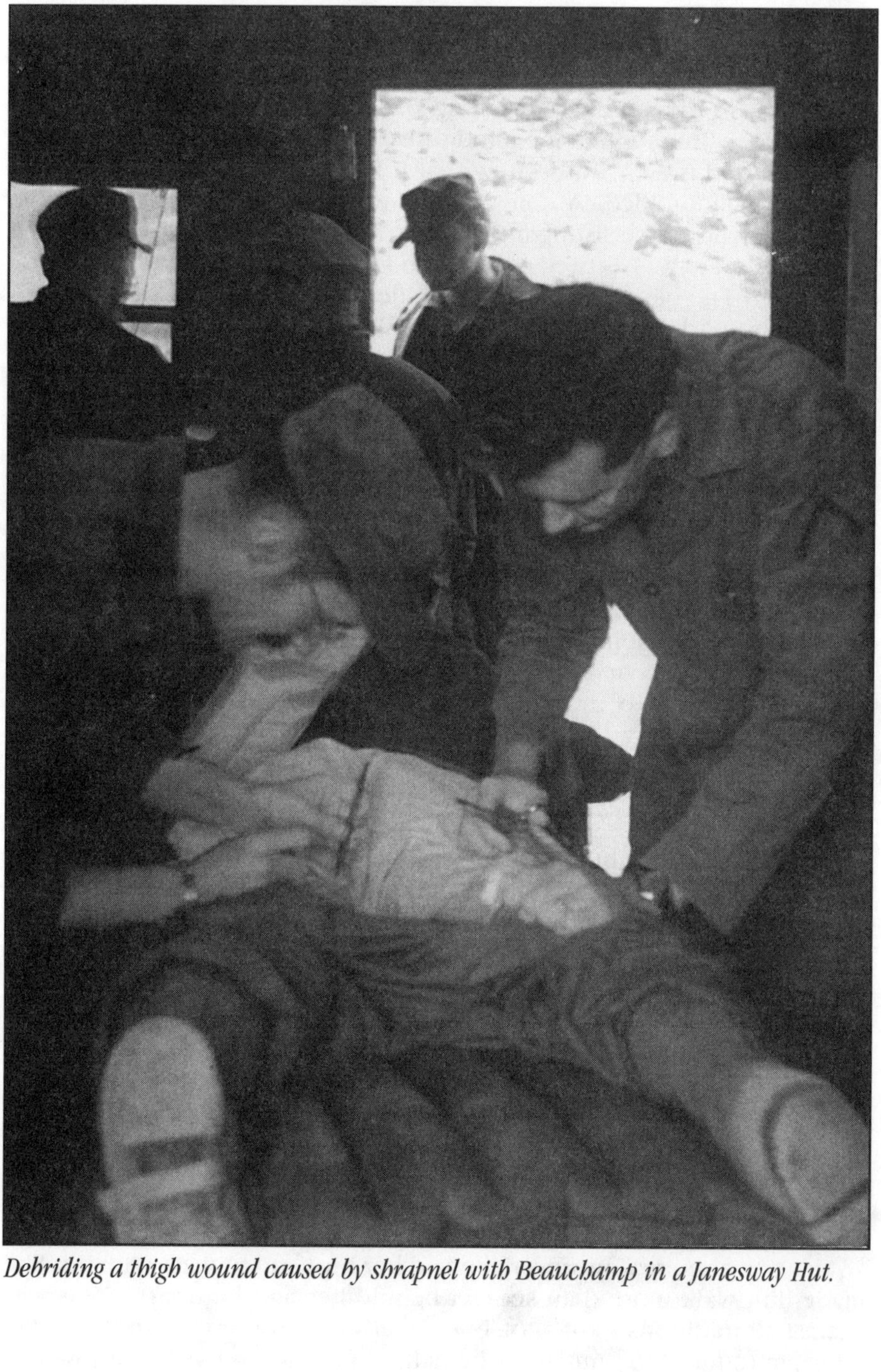

Debriding a thigh wound caused by shrapnel with Beauchamp in a Janesway Hut.

to a neighbor, Chipper Chapman's, farm to sell the bull's services.

Mae was out in front, as usual, with Seth and the bull behind by a good fifteen feet. Seth was holding onto the bull by a ring through its nose with a chain attached. What happened next is anyone's guess, for no one was a witness. Some thought it was only an accident, while others say Seth and Mae were having a rip-roaring fight and Seth let go of the bull on purpose, tired of being treated like a second class citizen.

Somehow the bull got free though, put his head down, and charged at Mae. She had been wearing a red shirt and khaki pants, the perfect target to attract the attention of a bull, and her swaying walk set it to charging.

Seth said he yelled out a warning to Mae, but as usual she ignored him. It probably wouldn't have mattered much even if she had listened to him for it was unlikely that she could have gotten out of the way in time.

The bull gored Mae in her right buttocks with his left horn and, according to Seth, threw her almost six feet into the air. Strangely enough the bull didn't repeat his attack. After throwing Mae, he continued on his way towards Chipper Chapman's farm. Seth was found kneeling next to his screaming and bleeding wife when a pickup truck came along and the driver and Seth somehow got Mae, screaming and swearing, into the back of the truck and headed for town.

It was the middle of the afternoon when the pickup truck arrived out in front of my office. Several people were in my waiting room waiting for me to attend to their various medical needs. All of them forgot their personal problems and scurried out to the truck to help carry Mae into my office, which was quite a sight. It wouldn't have been any easier for them if they had tried to carry the bull! But they succeeded and carefully steadied her on her stomach onto the examining/surgical table which was only 24 inches wide. Mae's backside was quite a bit wider than the table.

I examined her quickly. She had a very large laceration, had lost a lot of blood, and was still bleeding profusely. I had to stop the bleeding and decided it would be best if she went to a hospital. She said, in no uncertain terms, that we were not going to be able to get her to the hospital. She wouldn't hear of it. Not only her size, but her stubbornness was taurine. I was to fix her up here in the office or she was somehow going to get home. That left me with one option. I had to fix her up the best I could, here in my office.

I gave her a shot of penicillin and tetanus toxoid in her left, undamaged, backside and proceeded to repair the laceration. It took 53 stitches as recorded in my log. Mae didn't complain once I had injected a local anesthesia. She was going to be okay.

The people in the waiting room were again recruited to carry Mae. They loaded her into the pickup and she and Seth were off back to Chippenhook.

I returned to my office to gaze at the patients I had kept waiting. I expected to see some anger, some resentment, but there were no complaints. They were all amused, and chattering away enjoying all the excitement and conjecture. Most thought Mae had gotten what she deserved, at least a little, for putting poor Seth through hell every day. They thought it was about time he fought back, even if he had let the bull do his dirty work. Others insisted that it had to be an accident; even poor, tortured Seth wouldn't set a bull on his wife.

The talk went on around town for days. Only Seth and the bull knew the real truth about the matter, though, and neither one ever told.

Chapter Ten

HOME DELIVERY

The sun was high in the sky and a cool breeze was blowing, turning the fields into a welcome oasis from the stifling heat. The morning events around camp had been slow so Beauchamp, Rector and I decided to take a walk along the path that ran between the two large rice paddies. Beauchamp and Rector walked ahead of me, it was like being free in the mist of the chaos of war we had been experiencing. Beauchamp and Rector were like children again, kicking and pushing each other. I chuckled and then my heartbeat shifted in warning. I realized that if one of them strayed into the mine laden rice fields they could get us all blown to smithereens.

"Come on, you guys! Knock it off! You're going to get us all killed!" I yelled ahead in warning.

"It's okay, Doc. There is plenty of room in between the mines for a little fun," Beauchamp yelled, not even turning around as he pushed Rector to the left.

I opened my mouth to chastise them again when a shadow rose over the crest of the hills in front of us. All three of us froze, as we stared at the Russian-made MIG Fighter as it flew higher into the sky, its wing span blocking out the rays of the sun, the only darkness in the cloudless summer sky. We held our breaths. It seemed to glide, shifting its course to the right, then just as quickly it swooped to the left and headed straight for us.

Beauchamp and Rector dove for the dirt, I stood paralyzed in fascination and horror. It was like a monstrous steel bird of prey and we were its next victims. As the jet flew its course I stood straight in its path, thinking only briefly that when he started firing, I may have a chance to dive to one side, but I had to watch for as long as I could. My reflexes were as tight as bow strings. I watched as the jet soared closer, bearing down on me, no more than twenty feet off the ground. I couldn't move, I felt the sweat begin to trickle down between my shoulder blades. I waited for the first of the machine gun fire to start blasting at the path before me. No shots came, the plane kept flying straight for me. Absentmindedly I read the writing on the underbelly of the plane, its message was an inconceivable scribble written in a language I didn't understand. As it flew over me, its immense body and wings cast me into shadow.

I turned, as the sun shone upon me again, and watched the war bird swoop around and circle, heading back toward the north as if he had just caught the breeze that was to take him where he was going.

Slowly, through my clenched teeth, I let out the breath I didn't know I had been holding. It was over and for some unknown reason the pilot of that plane didn't fire on us. I silently gave thanks and turned my attention to my two comrades that were still face down in the dirt on the path in front of me.

"Hey, you guys," I yelled as I walked up to them, "get up out of the dirt. He is long gone now."

As I helped them both to their feet, they were still shaking. It was decided, without saying a word to one another, that we would keep walking ahead. We walked in complete silence. Our self-imposed censorship was our way to take in all that had just happened and try to find an answer to why that pilot didn't fire on us. We walked a long way, past the mine fields and all the way to the base of the hill, before any one of us uttered a word. It was Rector who asked aloud the question we all had been thinking.

"Hey, Doc, why didn't he fire on us?"

I shrugged. I had no idea. But I answered with a simple statement, "Maybe he was out of ammo."

The three of us sat down on a rock ledge which had been warmed by the sun, not saying anything and just glad to be alive. After a few minutes, Beauchamp turned to me and blurted out, "Hey, Doc, how about telling us another one of your Vermont stories?"

Grateful to him for changing the subject lingering in our minds, I gladly obliged. "Let's see now," I began, "there was one aspect of general practice I did not enjoy and I don't think anyone does - home deliveries."

Soon after arriving in town I was informed by another doctor at the hospital that there would be an occasional home delivery. He told me that if I fixed up a separate bag with obstetrical equipment in it that I would have no problem. Wrong. It took me one such adventure to realize that home deliveries were very much of a problem and no fun. These people were mostly from way out in the boonies where there was much inbreeding and many of them were transients. During my two years and three months as a general practitioner of medicine, I had a perfect record of never being paid for a home delivery. I thought $50 was a reasonable fee; I never even got a chicken or any vegetables.

A few weeks after I arrived in town there was a call from a man from Hubberton, which is exactly 13 miles northwest. "Hey, Doc, I got a woman going to have a baby out here. Can you come?"

"What's your name?"

"Guy Saunders."

"Guy, I don't know that area too well," I told him, "but do know where Hubberton Four Corners is located."

"OK, Doc, I'll meet you there."

Sure enough, he was at Hubberton Four Corners when I arrived. He was driving a beat-up 1942 Ford pickup truck. Somehow he knew it was me and waved for me to follow. Guy left the main dirt road and entered a lane which in turn was the entrance to a large field. I parked behind him and got out, fetched my obstetrical bag from the trunk, and we shook hands. Guy looked to be about 30 years old. I followed him up the steep grade across the field. I could see a shack more than a hundred yards the other side of this field.

"Guy, who's having the baby?" I asked.

"It's my housekeeper. I was living here alone until this past year when

I advertised for a housekeeper in the Rutland Herald." This transaction was evidently accomplished by the United States Postal Service for Guy did not have a telephone and for that matter, electricity either. He had called me from the general store at Hubberton Corners.

"Guy, why didn't you come in for prenatal examinations?"

"Uh...what's that?" he asked

"It's a checkup," I told him, "to see if there are going to be any problems with the delivery and to make certain that the woman and the baby are in good health."

"Doc, she was more than six months pregnant when she arrived here. I didn't have the heart to turn her away even though it's someone else's kid."

Just then, a dog came around the corner of the hut. I could tell by the look in his eyes, as he galloped in my direction, that he did not like me. I was just about to bolt when Guy quickly grabbed a snow shovel and started swinging. He clubbed the poor dog on the side of the head so hard it stopped him cold. I could almost see his eyes juggle around in his big shaggy head. The sound of the shovel hitting his skull was like a bell ringing as it resounded across the field and echoed down in the hollow. The dog shook his head, pulled his tongue back into his mouth and staggered around the side of the hut back where he had come from. I noticed he was wagging his tail. I guess any attention is better than none!

I opened the door of the shack and walked in ahead of Guy. There was one large room which he obviously used as living room, dining room and kitchen. A beat-up grand piano served as a dining room table. A couple of kitchen chairs, a couch and a pot-bellied stove completed the decor. I couldn't help wondering why Guy needed a housekeeper? These people were poor.

"Where's the patient, Guy?"

He opened a door across the room which I had not seen. It opened only part way for there was a bed in the way. I slid in sideways, turned around and saw Guy heading out the front door. He wasn't about to be any part of this "having a baby" business.

Inside this room was a metal-framed double bed which occupied most of the small room. A very pregnant young woman was on the bed. She looked real scared. She wasn't having contractions at the moment, so I sat on the side of the bed and introduced myself

"Hi, I'm Dr. Montgomery. I'm here to help you with your baby. What's your name?"

"Susan," she answered apprehensively.

"How old are you, Susan?"

"Nineteen."

"And where are you from?" I was hoping to relax her a little bit before we got to work.

"I've been wandering," she explained.

"Who's the father?" I asked.

"I don't know." She was not one for long explanations, I guess.

It wasn't long before the scared look left her face and she felt comfortable with me. Then she began with contractions and started to bear down. She made no sound or complaint

"Does it hurt, Susan?"

"Yes, it's getting a little bad."

"You can cry out all you want. Sometimes, it helps. Susan, you'd better take off your clothes and cover up with one of those blankets."

Back in those days and probably still today, patients were shaved and prepared with antiseptic solution prior to delivery. There was no chance to do this with the home delivery. The only other items in the room were two blankets, a stack of towels and a cardboard box. The bed had a metal headboard and fortunately no footboard, otherwise it would have been impossible to help with a delivery in this small room.

While Susan was taking off her clothes, I faced in the opposite direction, turned the cardboard box upside down, covered it with a towel and arranged the equipment in a neat row so that it would be handy during the delivery. The equipment consisted on a can of ether, an ether mask, umbilical tape, hemostats, scissors, rubber gloves and a set of outlet forceps which had been wrapped and sterilized.

"Now, Susan, I have to do an examination of you inside to see how the baby is coming." I put on a rubber glove and found that the cervix was two and a half fingers dilated which meant that she was fairly well along with her labor.

During the next two hours Susan and I got to know each other quite well, that is, in between contractions, which were up to one minute in duration by this time.

She was a primipara (first baby) by all signs and verified this when I asked her. With the first baby it is quite often necessary to do an episiotomy, which is making a skin cut in the back part of the vagina to allow the head to come out more easily and to prevent tearing of tissues. There were two ways to give anesthesia for this: local novocaine in the area, general open drop ether anesthesia, or both.

Soon her contractions were almost continuous. She let out a few yelps, but made much less noise than the average patient. As the head began to come into view, she did cry out quite a bit. I'm sure I would have, too!

"Come on, Susan, put your knees up and move down towards me."

In order to ease her pain, I put the mask over her face and dropped ether until she was quiet, and then ran down to the other end to see how things were going. After going back and forth several times, I made the cut following a few good whiffs of ether. She yelled out, but I didn't think she would remember the pain.

The baby presented LOA (left occiput anterior), which is the most common presentation and usually an easy delivery.

Out the baby came. I grabbed the baby's ankles and held her upside down. After cleaning the secretions from her mouth, I gave her a whack on the butt and she let out a cry.

"What is it?"

"A girl, Susan, and a beauty."

"Thanks, Doc," Susan was beaming brightly now.

I laid the baby down between her legs and held onto it with my left hand. The umbilical cord was still attached inside to the placenta (afterbirth). I began massaging the uterus through the abdomen with my left hand. Soon the placenta was delivered. The application of two clamps and a cut with scissors separated the baby from the placenta. The cord was tied next to the baby's bellybutton. I picked a novocaine syrette and catgut suture material from my bag and repaired the episiotomy. Lastly, a drop of silver nitrate went into the baby's eyes to counteract any potential infection. After wrapping the baby in a towel, I put it in Susan's arms and covered them both with a blanket. She smiled like only a new mother can, with every cell of her body. I borrowed one of their towels to wrap my equipment and placed this in my obstetrical bag.

Now, where was Guy? I found him sitting in the field about a hundred feet from the shack, just far enough so he could not hear the sounds of the delivery.

"Hey, Guy, I'll come back tomorrow and give you instructions as to Susan's and the baby's care."

"Doc, I have a woman neighbor coming in for a few days to care for them."

On my way home I vowed this would be my last home delivery. It wasn't.

The next day the mother and baby were doing well. A very fat farm woman had the shack cleaned and obviously had taken over. On my way to the car I mentioned that it would be necessary for me to fill out a birth certificate and they should have some names ready for me in a couple of days.

"By the way, Doc. I asked Susan to marry me and she said yes. A preacher is coming out in a few days. Can you make out that certificate saying we're married?"

I don't know whether this was legal or not, but I did it anyway. Also, I never got any pay for the delivery, as I mentioned before, but then, it never seemed to bother me much.

As for the Russian-made MIG fighter not firing on us, I later heard that someone in Washington had made a deal with the North Koreans, or Chinese Communists to the effect that if we would not bomb above the Yalub River then they would not strafe our troops with their jets. Some politician had probably saved our lives that day.

Chapter Eleven

TWINS

My next story to the corpsmen about my general practice days was about twins.

The treatment of urological diseases was rather primitive during my days of general practice. For example, cystitis or inflammation of the bladder was treated using a dye called pyridium and sulfonamides. When it didn't respond to this, which was quite often, I would catheterize the patient and instill into the bladder a solution known as argerol, which is a silver protein. This somehow would decrease the bacterial count and also relieve their symptoms of pain, spasm and frequent urination. This is more frequent in the female than the male. If you can figure this out, give me a call or write me a letter.

Prostatitis was a frequent complaint. The symptoms here were difficulty and burning on urination and often a discharge from the urethra. Penicillin and sulfa drugs were of some use here but prostatic massage was often necessary. Repeated prostatic massage at least twice a week over a period of many weeks was required before this disease came under control. Fortunately, there were not too may cases of prostatitis in the rural country, otherwise I think I would have quit general practice right there. The patient would come in, take down his pants and bend over. I would, with a rubber glove on my right hand, insert the index finger into his rectum and massage the prostate, as I remember, about 20 times on each side of the prostate, which has two lobes. While doing this, material would most often leak out of his urethra and onto his pants, or a gauze that I had given him.

Rubber gloves were not disposable as they are now. I would, after completing the massage, go out into the sterilizing room where I had a special sink to wash these gloves with soap and water, then sterilizing solution. Following this, they would be placed in a rack to be sterilized. Then they had to be hung to dry. Rubber gloves were relatively expensive in those days and we used the same technique following surgical procedures in the hospital. It seemed there was always a nurse in the utility room cleaning and sterilizing rubber gloves. There is a real art to this, and I bet not many doctors or nurses would know how to perform this task today. Everything now is disposable and contributes to medical waste as well as polluting our environment.

Obstetrics wasn't too bad except for home deliveries and unwanted or illegitimate pregnancies. Prenatal care was important. Of utmost importance was to make certain that the mother had sufficient and the right type of nourishment for both her and the baby. Office visits consisted of measuring their pelvis, making sure that they were anatomically OK for a vaginal delivery. I had excellent training and experience in obstetrics which gave me a great deal of confidence, which I suspect is nine-tenths of the battle. My professor of obstetrics gave me this confidence and one word of advice, and that was, "Never use anything other than outlet forceps for a delivery and you will get along OK."

For the most part, the pregnant women would give me sufficient warning so that I could either drive them to or meet them at the hospital and stay with them until the baby was born. After arriving at the hospital, I followed them carefully by checking the degree of dilation of the cervix. When the head or the part being delivered first drops into the pelvis, the cervix, or bottom of the uterus, begins to dilate. Dilation of the cervix is measured by "finger widths" rather than inches or centimeters. It's a measurement of feel rather than sight. When the cervix is about 3-4 fingers dilated, and the contractions are less than one minute apart, it is time to get into action.

My technique for "painless delivery" was to use a "dropped" spinal anesthesia. I would sit the patient up on the edge of the bed and she would hug the nurse who faced her from the opposite side. This way it was very easy to perform a spinal tap. Once I was certain I was in the spinal canal, I would instill a small amount of local anesthetic which was combined with a hypertonic (heavy) solution which would drop in the spinal column and anesthetize only the pelvic region. Thus, it would be necessary for her to remain sitting for a few minutes to make certain that this droppage occurred. As she was sitting, she would describe the anesthesia occurring in the area in and around her vagina. Using this technique, a patient could contract her abdominal muscles for bearing down and the delivery could be accomplished rather painlessly and easily. Most often during a delivery I performed an episiotomy, which is, as previously mentioned, an incision made in the perineum between the rectum and the vagina. This increases the outlet opening and prevents stretching and tearing of the muscles. Most deliveries occurred during the night. Don't ask me why, I just don't know.

You could always tell when a doctor had been up the night before with a long labor for he was dragging his butt and had bags under his eyes.

There's a couple of deliveries that I just have to tell you about. During the spring of the second year of my practice, two of my former high school classmates came to me when they were several months pregnant. I was thrilled, astonished and flattered that they were going to let me deliver their babies.

One girl lived on a farm about 5 miles outside of town. This was a beautiful farm which was run by her father and three brothers. Her mother was an excellent cook, and I often stopped in for breakfast when I was out that way on an early house call. This was Marcia. Maggie, the second classmate, grew up on the same street as I, only six houses apart. I went to a high school dance with her one time.

I calculated from their last menstrual periods that they were both due in August. They both had extremely large bellies but had not gained excessive weight elsewhere. I suspected both of them that they either had an excessive amount of amniotic fluid or had twins. No ultrasound in those days. I at least imagined in both that I could hear two distinct heartbeats with my fetal stethoscope.

Maggie was first. I got a call from her husband about 10 o'clock in the evening and went to her house for an examination. The three of us drove to the hospital. Her amniotic sac ruptured at about 1 a.m.This is referred to more commonly as "her water broke." Her cervix was fully dilated shortly thereafter so I sat her up and gave her a dropped spinal anesthesia. I delivered the first baby after performing an episiotomy without event and started to massage her uterus to encourage delivery of the placenta. Her uterus was still enormous. Not until then was I sure that there was another baby. Her contractions continued and she delivered the second baby within an hour. They were identical twin boys.

Two weeks later, Marcia delivered in the same fashion. This time I was sure I could hear two heartbeats and was ready for the second twin. The delivery was uneventful. Marcia had beautiful twin girls. After they were born, I was checking the baby girls for any defects and almost cut my finger on two lower incisors which had already erupted. I was more cautious when examining the second twin. Sure enough, she also had two lower incisors. Somehow the press got a hold of this information and the front page of the next morning's paper read, "Identical Twin Girls Born with Teeth!"

Somehow, I think Marcia was a little disappointed and envious of Maggie's twin boys, for at least in those days, males were more desirable than females for continuation of the family farm.

Sixteen years later, in June, I received a letter from the principal of the high school inviting me to be graduation speaker. My two sets of twins were graduating from high school. Our pictures were on the front page of the local newspaper the following day.

Beauchamp and Rector were still listening to me.

"That's it, my friends," I told them.

Along with assisting in the birth of a baby comes a deep satisfaction of being part of initiating a new life, a huge contrast to being in combat where lives are being taken away or even worse, maimed so that a beautiful young body is altered to such a degree that further existence is a torture or a misery.

Chapter Twelve

MORE GENERAL PRACTICE

One day when we were working in the sickbay tent, the corpsmen asked me to tell them yet another general practice story. "Well, guys, before telling you the next general practice story, I must describe to you a bit about the marble industry."

The marble is cut from the quarry in the shape of large cubes or blocks. These measure anywhere from ten to fifteen feet in all dimensions and even larger for special projects. These pieces of marble are lifted from the quarry by a large derrick and then transferred to a flatbed railroad car which in turn transports the marble to its place of storage. When the car reaches the storage area, two large loops of cable are placed around the block of marble and it is lifted from the railroad flatbed to its temporary resting place by a huge crane. Hundreds and hundreds of these large pieces of marble are stacked one on top of the other, three layers high, for a distance of more than 100 yards. The blocks of marble remain stacked until they are needed for some project, when they are again lifted by the crane onto the flatbed railroad car. They are then transferred to the mill where they are sawed into the desired sized pieces.

As you can well imagine, many of us as children had secret hiding places, or as we called them, caves, in among these large blocks of marble. Several kids of the same age would have one of these caves as their hide-out for storage of secret items such as pea shooters, bb guns, occasionally a few cigarettes, and the like.

They also were a very fine shelter for tramps. In case you don't know, a tramp is an outdoors person who prefers to live a life of poverty either by himself or with other tramps. They wander continuously. In the city, we refer to them as "street people."

One evening at about 10 p.m., I got a call from the sheriff telling me that there was a man who was probably dead up near the main quarry stockpile. I met the sheriff downtown and we rode up to the main quarry in his car. On the way he said, "Doc, I don't know whether I should have called you or Father Orzek. Fred and Sam are up there in the vicinity and drunk as usual." Fred and Sam were a couple of town drunks who did enough part time work to keep them in booze and didn't get into too much trouble. Sam didn't have any toes. He passed out a couple of winters before that time and when they found him, all of his toes were severely frostbitten and needed to be amputated.

As I remember it was a cold autumn evening. The moon was not out so it was very dark. The sheriff had a flashlight and we fumbled our way among the alleyways formed by the blocks, listening to an occasional vocal utterance from either Fred or Sam. We finally reached them and they were sitting on a marble ledge with a candle between them for illumination and playing cards. I suspect they were playing a game called Bid 45, which was the favorite game of many people in town.

"Hey, Doc, you ain't gonna do this guy much good. I think he's a goner."

Looking down directly below them, I saw the recumbent figure of a man lying and covered with newspaper except for his head. I do believe that newspapers are the universal blanket for tramps, or at least it was in those days. When I first looked at him I thought they were right and that he was dead. I did, however, detect a faint carotid pulse and shallow breathing. An examination of his chest with my stethoscope confirmed this and also that his lungs were congested and that he probably had pneumonia. His blood pressure was 75/50.

"Tom, I think we had better get him to the hospital. He is not going to last much longer here."

Sam, who was a fairly well educated man and had done well until the booze got the best of him, said, "Doc, let him stay there. You take him inside and give him a bath and you'll kill him for sure!" At that point Fred gave the sign of the cross.

"Come on Fred and Sam, you guys seem sober enough. Give us a hand."

"No need, Doc," was Sam's reply. They had no intention of having their drinking and card playing interfered with.

Tom and I had to drag this poor tramp, who by the way was quite ripe, a considerable distance before we reached the sheriff's car. For the most part he was unconscious, giving an occasional moan. We transported him to the hospital where I talked another general practitioner into taking over his care. This other doctor was waiting around for a delivery and didn't seem to mind.

Tom and I got back to the main street of West Rutland at about 12:30 a.m. I was just walking over to my car when someone yelled from Joe's restaurant and bar, "Hey, Doc, come on over here! We need you!" My first thought was to keep walking for I knew that by this time, everyone at Joe's was fairly inebriated. Ah, what the hell, maybe they do need me.

As I walked into Joe's establishment, which by the way was used very occasionally for eating, but most often for drinking, there were only three people present: Joe, Marie the barmaid, and her husband.

"Come on in, Doc, and have a drink on the house! How would you like a boilermaker?"

"Joe, you know I can't drink unless I'm out of town on vacation. What's up? It's late and I'm getting a little tired."

Joe had been a patient of mine ever since I had begun practice. He was a diabetic which I had in good control. He also had a leg ulcer which I had been treating rather unsuccessfully for the past few months. As far as I could make out from my books and talking with the other doctors, painting the ulcer with gentian violet and then sprinkling on aluminum dust was the best treatment to stimulate healing. It had reduced in size slightly and showed no signs of secondary infection.

"Doc, how about looking at my ulcer."

"Joe, you know you have an appointment to see me next week."

"Yeah, but this thing is really hurting me, Doc. Take a look at it."

He pulled up his pantleg and there had been no change in the ulcer. I knew it would do no good to argue with him so I went back to my car, got my medical bag and painted the ulcer with some gentian violet.

I didn't have any aluminum powder with me.

I closed my bag and was about to leave when Marie, who was more than slightly inebriated said, "Doc, take a look at my hernia!" At this point she proceeded to remove her slacks and underwear which dropped to her ankles. There she stood naked from the waist down! I can imagine what someone looking in the window would think about this performance.

I examined her direct inguinal hernia, washed my hands, and took Joe up on his offer for a boilermaker.

There were no further calls that night and I slept well.

I remember Grandpa Salen. Everyone in town called him Grandpa. I suspect the reason for this was that he was always out, visible, doing his chores, either taking care of his laying hens or working in his garden. He always looked old, even when I remember him when I was a kid, but with a very kindly face. I never saw him without the Grandpa attire: a workshirt, bib overalls, boots and a soft hat. His daughter, Margaret, was our third grade school teacher and had long given up trying to dress him up so that he could go to church on Sunday. Probably about twice a year, Grandpa would find himself a bottle of whiskey. I think he bought the cheap stuff which was a homemade brew made in the basement of some of the Polish immigrant's homes. I am told that this is pretty potent stuff and a few ounces would knock you to nowhere for sometime. When I came back to West Rutland and started in general practice, Grandpa was real old, but he still was well enough to "enjoy" his binge drinking. One time, Grandpa's absence extended to more than one week and I became concerned for his whereabouts and welfare. I met his daughter, Ethel, in the post office and asked, "Where's Grandpa?"

"Oh, William," she answered, "he's not been feeling well. I wish you would come by and see him. He's been in bed for nearly a week."

That evening after office hours, I drove up to the Salen house and went in to examine Grandpa, who also called me William. He had had a minor stroke after one of his three day binges and had been, for the most part, lying in bed. He had not been drinking enough fluids, so he was dehydrated. He was having a problem with both his waterworks and his alimentary tract. Grandpa had not moved his bowels for more than one week. I went back to the office and got an intravenous solution so I could counteract his dehydration. Disempactment was painful as per usual.

It took me about two weeks of daily housecalls to get Grandpa back in shape. Finally, I found him sitting in the chair looking out the window when I arrived. You know, almost always I brought my black dog along with me in the front seat of my car when making house calls, especially at night. This dog's name was "Alexis Ebony". I called her Ex-Lax for short. She was a very sweet dog, and the only thing she ever did wrong was to pee on the post office floor every time anyone would try to pet her, which was every time we went to the post office.

Grandpa kept looking out at my car and squinting. He pulled the curtain aside and put his head right up against the glass and said, "William! You don't have your wife with you today!"

All this time he thought Ex-Lax was my wife. I guess his vision wasn't too good either.

"I left her home, Grandpa."

Grandpa got all better and tended to his laying hens and his garden again. A few months later, however, he had another stroke and died. Everyone misses Grandpa.

"And that," I added, "is the end of my general practice stories."

Chapter Thirteen

PROHIBITION

The air around us stood still in the heat. We had sought shelter inside the bunker taking refuge on the cool dirt floor from the onslaught of stifling temperatures and the ever closer incoming shells. The enemy fire and our side's retaliation beat out a destructive tattoo. The sounds of war carried for miles, and at times it seemed as if it reached up to the heavens, shaking the moon and the millions of stars in the clear summer night sky. The reverberations of battle surrounded us and like the unforgiving heat, it seemed to enter our pores.

Strangely, I was not afraid. I had friends around me, my fellow marines, plus I had heard these sounds before and experienced enemy shelling many times and at closer range. I guess, in a morbid way I had gotten used to it.

Actually, I was glad I wasn't alone. When I first arrived in Korea and assumed my duties as a combat medical officer I realized that if I played it by the book and created a rank barrier between me and the enlisted personnel my time in Korea could be a very lonely experience. Combat is lonely enough without segregating yourself from those you work with. So, early on I decided I wouldn't stand on protocol. I made it a point, part of my job, to get to know each and every one of my corpsmen, their names, what part of the States they came from, and everything they wanted to tell me I was glad to listen to. More than once I heard that I wasn't like those other officers, but a regular guy, and working with me had been more of a collaborative effort than just an "asshole" officer giving orders like he was "dictator". Each time I heard a marine say that to me it made me happy and I knew my decision to go against the rules wasn't for naught. Of course, if I were a line officer it would have been different. I made many good friends and, gratefully, I never wanted for someone to talk to. I know, in a way, I had made my stay in Korea that much more difficult. Each time a friend was wounded or killed, I mourned. In one month alone I lost every corpsmen, either killed or wounded, except for my two "body guards", Beauchamp and Rector. I grieved for each of my friends more than if they had been just a bunch of serial numbers. But if I had a choice, I would not trade a minute of the friendships I had made to save my heart some of the pain.

We had a bottle of booze and we were passing it around. By the way, it was against the rules to drink hard stuff with the enlisted personnel, but I did it anyway. The bourbon bottle made me think of Adam Polinski, so I told the guys about Adam.

One night in late August, I woke up with a start from a sound sleep at 11:30 p.m. It was warm and all the stars were out. I clearly remember the time since I was looking down at my first wrist watch which had hands and numbers that glowed in the dark. They don't make those anymore. My parents had given it to me for my ninth birthday a few days previously. It soon became obvious that I had been awakened by a very loud dialogue among several people out in the street in front of one of our neighbor's houses. This was unusual, for we were still living in a small house on the main street which had quite a bit of traffic noise during the night, and I had become a sound sleeper. This noise was different. People were yelling and swearing. I got out of bed and peered through the open window to see Mrs. Polinski yelling at a man in a white suit who was handcuffing her husband, Adam. Joe, our town sheriff, was also present, but not doing much other than looking on. He looked embarrassed.

Why were they arresting Adam? Such a nice man. The Polinski's didn't have any children of their own, so they were like Aunt and Uncle to all us kids. Adam worked for the Vermont Marble Company and was a carpenter. He had taught me to make the skipper, which is the snow vehicle that I have described previously. It is made from a board wide enough to sit on, about five feet long, with barrel staves underneath for runners. As you remember, Franklin Delano Roosevelt's CCC (Civil Conservation Corps) along with the WPA had come into town and built us a beautiful toboggan slide down the side of one of the mountains that surrounded our town. I still wonder why someone has not acquired a patent for this device and manufactured it. It is an ingenious apparatus for gliding on the snow. The idea had come from Poland with Adam.

Adam was hauled off in the man-in-the-white-suit's car. Joe followed in his car. Mrs. Polinski was still yelling and crying as they drove away. All of this bothered me quite a bit because I considered Adam to be one of my close friends. I guess I stayed awake, off and on, most of the night. The next morning I was out of bed bright and early as usual. (My brother used to sleep until 10 a.m. or later during the summer.) During breakfast I asked my mother why Adam had been arrested. She pretended not to understand me. My mother was deaf but read lips beautifully. I suspect deaf people do, on occasion, take advantage of their disability and use this ploy when they do not want to answer a question. I tried my father next. He said it had something to do with prohibition and that we best not talk about it. I didn't know what the word 'prohibition' meant, so I dropped the subject.

After breakfast I went out in the backyard. Even at the age of nine years, I can remember the delight bursting out into a warm summer morning in the country. I had about 15 hens at the time. Hens, you know, are kind of stupid, but on the other hand, they seemed to know me, or at least associated my presence with food and water which I gave to them twice a day. I gathered up the eggs in a basket and brought them back into the house where I gave them to my mother. I always walked back from the hen house, at least ever since the day I was running and tripped with a large number of eggs in the basket. Not only did every egg break, but there was raw egg in my hair, on my face, and clothes. I'm sure you get the picture. My mother didn't laugh at me to avoid hurting my feelings, but told me it would be best that I did not run with eggs anymore. My father had gone to work and my mother was doing things in the kitchen, so after cleaning up I went into the living room and took the dictionary down from the shelf. After 'prohibition' it had "a law prohibiting the manufacture or sale of alcoholic beverage."

Thinking that some of the older boys would know more about this, I headed for the corner drug store. As per usual, there were a bunch of older boys talking on the steps. These steps were not like most steps, for they were more than 15 feet wide and led to a large porch and the entrance door to the drug store.

"You guys know why Adam Polinski was arrested last night?"

"What? Are you stupid or something?" Henry said, "Old Adam was making booze in his basement, and has been for years! This is the third time they've hauled him off to jail. He'll probably stay there for a while this time. The Feds came back early this morning and took all the whiskey he had made. You must have been sleeping."

"How does he make it?" I asked.

"From potatoes, like they do back in Poland. You can bet your sweet little ass he has made a lot of money and has it stashed away in his basement somewhere."

I felt sorry for Adam, but guess I shouldn't have. He was breaking the law.

Shortly thereafter I began waking up at night again. Maybe I wouldn't have if I didn't have booze and prohibition on my mind. This time it was cars racing by the house late at night. Most of the time it was just one car, or maybe two cars together. Then I became aware of definite pattern. The first car, or cars, would go by at high speed, and then there would be a hiatus of five to ten minutes, and a second car would whiz by the house. It became quite obvious that the second car was in pursuit of the first.

I thought about this for a long time, but didn't talk about it until one day when my father was in a real good mood.

"Dad, do you hear cars going by the house real fast during the night?"

"Yes."

"Why are they going so fast and what are they doing? There's some real strange things going on around here, and I think I should know a little bit about them. Also, they took Adam away to jail two weeks ago, and he's not home yet."

He broke down and told me all about prohibition. He said it started in 1920 long before I was born, by the 18th Amendment and Volstead Act, and that it was becoming a serious social problem.

Adam Polinski is a bootlegger and has been making home brew in his basement for many years. The liquor dealers, or rum runners as they call them, come down country roads from Canada where they purchase the liquor. Most often they do this at night and blast through border checkpoints. Sometimes the federal agents spot them and it becomes a cops and robbers chase. The rum runners know the back roads all the way from Canada down through Vermont and New Hampshire on the way to Boston and New York City where they sell the liquor to a "speakeasy."

He showed me a map and pointed to some of the various routes that skirted cities such as St. Albans, Burlington, and Middlebury, Vermont.

They often came down a back road on the east side of Lake Bomoseen and then hit Route 4, which is the main drag going by our house.

Actually, prohibition was a very interesting period in the United States history. Many states had adopted prohibition before 1920. Why they passed prohibition is a very complex question. It certainly didn't stop people from drinking liquor. The answer to why prohibition was repealed is quite simple. The Wall Street crash of 1929, and the Depression which followed in the 1930's, led to its repeal in 1933. Hunger was a far more elegant proponent than any speech against its repeal.

The relationship of prohibition and the Roaring Twenties is not entirely clear. Certainly drinking became more fashionable than ever and led to a decline in social behavior. The "speak easy" now replaced the saloon. The term "speakeasy" originated in Ireland as "speak softly shop." In the1920's, a new phrase came into the English language to describe the smuggling of liquor into the United States, "Rum Running". Smuggling provided the surest way to obtain liquor at a high quality. Travelers returning from Canada with liquor which was not concealed were not fined, but the liquor was confiscated. If they concealed liquor, they were fined $2 a bottle for beer, and $5 for wine, as well as losing the liquor. Men concealed liquor in belts and pockets; women concealed it in bloomers, corsets and false busts. Hay and lumber were common camouflage for liquor. Probably the most common method was automobiles with secret compartments.

A Rum Runner could buy good scotch in Canada for $4/bottle and sell it for $18 in New York City. He could make from $600 to $1200 a trip, and make two trips a week in summer and one in winter, providing the roads were clear of snow. His yearly income would be comparable to more than a million dollars today!

By 1932, Canada had increased its importation of liquor from England by six times. Hundreds of thirsty people would travel every Friday night or Saturday morning by train from New York City and New England to Montreal or Quebec.

In 1914, more than one third of the Federal government's revenue came from liquor trade, and after prohibition this was lost. By 1932, millions of people were unemployed. In prosperous times, voters tolerated the inefficiency and the one and a half billion dollars a year loss in liquor taxes. Repeal would reopen jobs for people in distilleries, winepresses, breweries, and liquor stores, bars and the like. Prohibition brought about more corruption in city government. During prohibition, bootleggers, gangsters, and racketeers made all the money that had previously been made for the government by liquor tax. There was no way that the prohibition law could be enforced. Even the medical profession got into the act. It has been calculated that 10 million prescriptions for more than 1 million gallons of alcohol were issued every year of prohibition. One half of these were fraudulent.

Three months later Adam came home and went back to work. This was the end of his bootlegging and the end of my story to the guys in a bunker somewhere in Western Korea along the 38th parallel.

Chapter Fourteen
ORDERS

A tour of duty in the United States Army in World War II as a private first class had not been to my liking, but little did I know that this training would be invaluable to me in the not too distant future.

Following my graduation from medical school, I decided to join the Navy Reserve as a lieutenant junior grade. My Reserve status continued during my 27 months of General Practice in West Rutland, Vermont. At this point, I received an invitation from the United States Navy to assume active duty. It was late summer, 1950. The Korean War was in its infancy and they needed doctors.

I received a tremendous outpouring of support from many of the patients. Some of them offered to make inquiries on my behalf in an attempt to defer my call to service, but I thought, "Why put off the inevitable," and graciously declined their offers.

After a week or so, since most of the people at that time still had the spirit of World War II, they accepted the thought of my leaving and got together a surprise party in the form of a big dance in a country barn.

The barn itself was a vision to behold. It was immaculate and festive with a Guernsey cow watching over the entrance. There were ribbons and bows adorning the inside, polka and square dancing, and a variety of Polish and American food. It seemed as though the whole town showed up. The party went on well into the wee hours of the morning. I truly believe this was the greatest honor of my life.

All too soon I left the town of my youth and the mountains I called home to report to the United States Navy Shipyard, Portsmouth, New Hampshire for my first tour of active duty. The shipyard occupies a small island which was connected to Kittery, Maine by a bridge. The main activities of the base were to construct and repair submarines and to house the United States Marine Corps Prison. My duty spot was a beautifully constructed brick hospital which was exactly the same design as the Naval hospitals at Chelsea, Massachusetts, Newport, Rhode Island and Portsmouth, Virginia.

On the day of my arrival, I interviewed with Captain Pinner, who was the Skipper of the hospital.

"Doctor, I run a tight ship. I am sure you will enjoy your tour of duty at Portsmouth Navy Hospital. I see you have been in General Practice. Have you had any training in Ear, Nose and Throat?" he asked.

"Yessir," I answered, "I had quite a bit during my internship and some extra training prior to entering General Practice. I have performed tonsillectomies and other Ear, Nose and Throat operations during my General Practice."

"Fine, then. I'll make you Chief of Eye, Ear, Nose and Throat", he informed me.

"Captain Pinner, I have had very little experience with eye disease and its treatment," I confessed.

He nodded. "OK, Doctor Montgomery. I am going to send you for two weeks of TAD (Temporary Additional Duty) at the Chelsea Navy Hospital under Captain Brown for a refresher course in ophthalmology."

After a "Yessir," and a salute, I went to my quarters to prepare for two weeks in Boston. During these next two weeks, I didn't see the light of day. My days were occupied with Captain Brown and his staff, my evenings were filled with study. I found the Captain was an excellent teacher but a real grouch.

Talk about a big frog in a little pond. Back in Portsmouth I had it made with my Department of Eye, Ear, Nose and Throat, which occupied the entire end of the hospital's first floor, and it was surrounded by excellent views in three directions. Under my command there were four corpsmen, all who had experience with eye, ear, nose and throat diseases and their treatments. The Chief Hospital Corpsman was an optometrist who graciously continued my education with refracting and the management of eye disease. (A chief in the navy is equivalent to a master sergeant in the army). I was immediately busy treating all sorts of problems. I even got to deliver an occasional baby when I was on call for the evening. This was only one day a week. My other evenings were free. What a contrast to General Practice!

I had never heard the word "comeshaw" before arriving at Portsmouth. Comeshaw is a real word and means "expression of thanks". As a medical officer, I was in a perfect position to practice the art of comeshaw, in order to obtain favors and supplies related to my hobby of wood carving. Navy Captains, equivalent to a full Army Colonel) and Chiefs are the best sources for these activities. For example, I comeshawed a supply of beautiful Idaho pine wood and used it to make a large sea chest. After dovetailing this wood into the form of a rectangular box, I sawed the top off. The metal shop provided me with a stainless steel piano-type hinge that ran the length of the whole chest. I then obtained wood to attach around the lid, which I carved into a rope and a square knot in the front as a handle. The metal shop constructed a stainless steel support for me that could be placed invisibly beneath this knot. On one end of the chest I carved a Spanish galley in full sail, and on the other, the Marine Corps emblem. On the front I carved a scale model of a submarine (the Tench) on which I had some training while at Portsmouth. The top of the chest was inlaid with a collection of rare woods from around the world. This sea chest, which I trust will be handed down for many generations, was made possible by a few kind words to and favors for my captain and chief patients - comeshaw.

I found that during my stay, having the United States Marine Corps prison nearby had it ups and its downs. It was somewhat depressing to see so many young men in trouble. It was one of the perks when one day while I was working in my office, an officer, who was about my age and size, came in for treatment of a sinus infection. I noted that he had been a lieutenant senior grade, my rank, and was in prison for the illicit selling of promotions to unlisted men. He seemed like a fairly nice fellow and I figured he was a wheeler and dealer so I asked him what he had done with his uniform. I had only purchased one set of blues when I entered the navy and I needed to purchase another. He immediately offered to sell me three sets of blues and one set of dress whites for only one hundred dollars. What a deal!

Possibly, one of the most interesting things that occurred during my stay at Portsmouth was my introduction to the submarine. I did have some training on the U.S.S. Tench, which was about the same size as a German World War II U-Boat. To this basic submarine structure, both a sonar and snorkel apparatus was added. Submariners are, without exception, superhuman. They are hand picked for compatibility. The first day aboard I was told that if a "bad apple" turned up while out at sea, he was immediately dropped on the first land sighted with shelter, and supplied with food, if necessary, to last him a few days. On a crew as close knit as this, one bad apple could spoil the whole barrel.

Every member of the 78 man crew played cribbage and I soon regained my skills with this game. Over all it was an exciting experience for me to learn about the details of submarine activity. Using the toilet in a sub was a real trick. If you made the slightest mistake you were apt to get it back in your face. It was a thrill to sneak up on ships using the periscope and to see how torpedoes were loaded and fired. The Skipper let me participate in these activities. There was one aspect of the submarine which I did not at all like. Occasionally, when we would go to a depth of greater than 600 feet, and if the pressure did not equalize, I experienced a severe pain in my ears and frontal sinuses. I don't remember any pain worse than this during my life thus far. I can only describe it as being similar to the pressure which occasionally occurs when descending in an airplane too rapidly, multiplied by ten. I swear I thought my head was going to explode during one of these episodes.

The navy is probably the most dignified of all branches of the service, especially when it comes to dining. Almost without exception, whether it be breakfast, lunch, or dinner, Naval officers sit at a table covered with a tablecloth and are provided with cloth napkins and silverware. I suspect this is a carry-over from the British Navy. I enjoyed my stay at Portsmouth and made many new friends.

I was having lunch in the Officer's Mess when one of the corpsmen came in and whispered, "The Skipper wants to see you, stat." Somehow, everyone at the table knew what was coming, but no one said anything.

I meandered into the Skipper's office, knocked, walked inside and saluted. He stood up, which struck me as unusual, saluted back and cleared his throat. His voice was clear but had an undercurrent of emotion as he told me why he summoned me.

"I have some orders for you, Bill." I knew that his use of my first name and by the expression on his face, that fate had severed the thread holding the sword that hangs over the head of every navy doctor, corpsman and Chaplain. As he told me my orders, I was no longer just a navy doctor, but I was now attached to the Fleet Marine Force. I was now a marine and I was bound for the Orient. As if in a daze, when he dismissed me, I "yessired", saluted, did an about face, departed from his office and walked slowly, mechanically back to my office.

I sat at my desk in stunned silence. Fleet Marine Force Duty was infrequently discussed among the officers and the corpsmen. We just didn't want to think of it and we didn't want to jinx ourselves by mentioning it. I was the first man to get FMF orders since I had arrived at Portsmouth. Two weeks before, I had gotten word that a former medical school classmate of mine, Lieutenant Senior Grade William Flood, had received sea duty orders for the west coast. I should have seen it coming. I should have expected that, with my previous training, I would have been called for duty with the marines.

Word of my orders spread like wildfire through out the hospital. Tension and apprehension hit a fevered pitch among most of my fellow doctors and corpsmen. One of the men took the news as a sure sign of

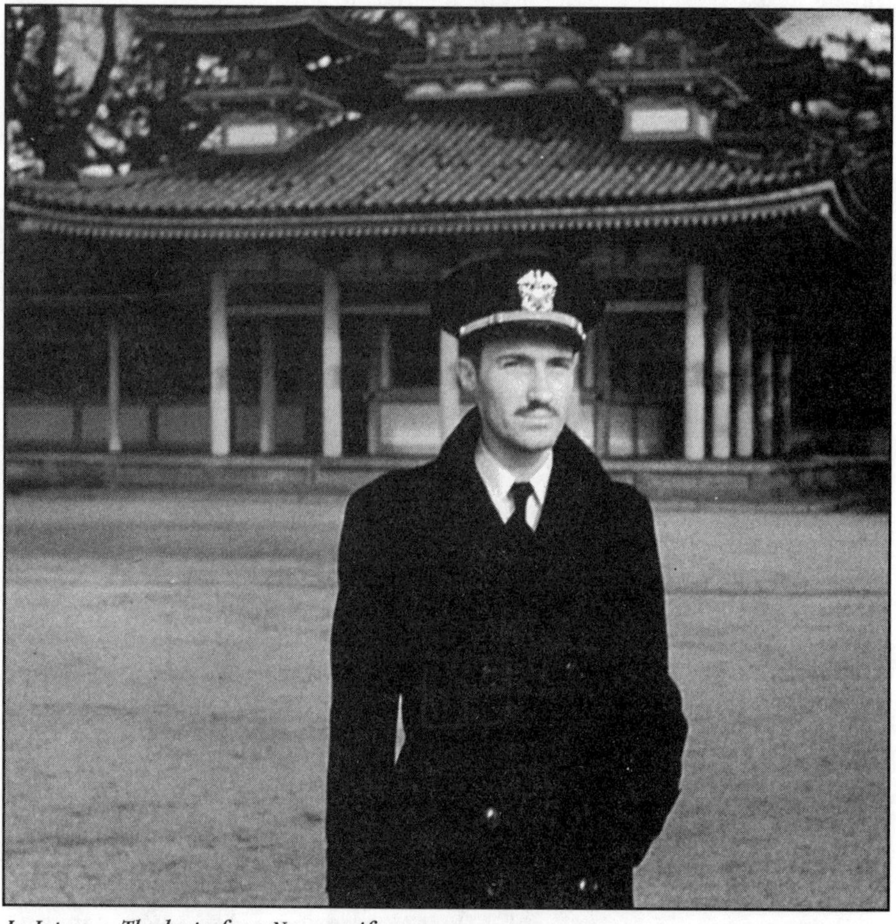

In Japan – The last of my Navy uniform.

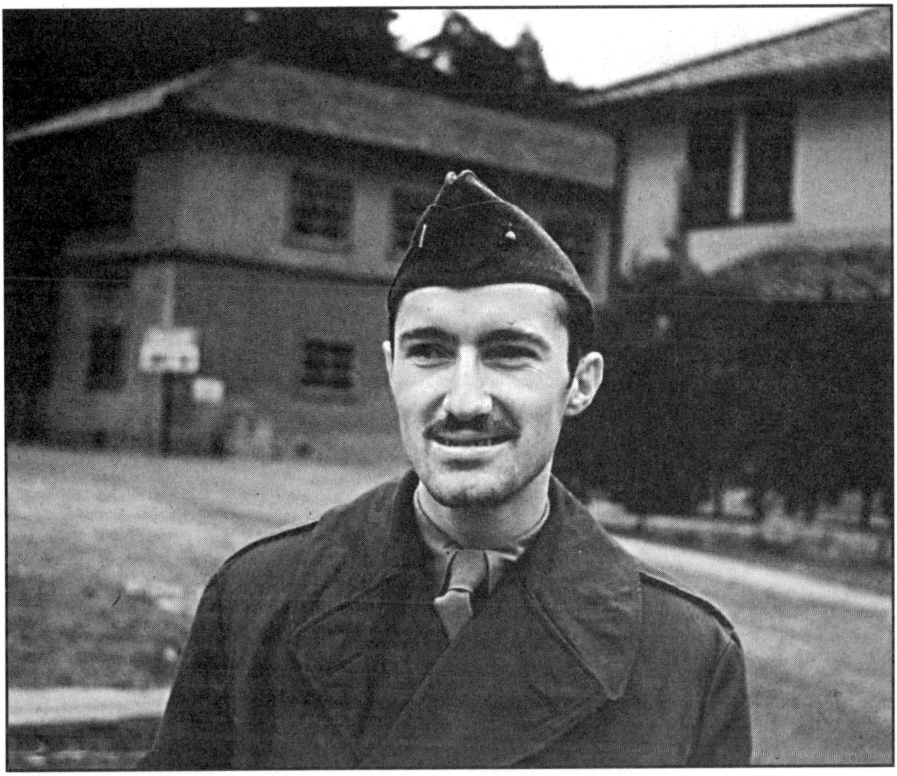

Into Marine uniform–Lieutenant Senior Grade U.S. Navy Reserve to 1st Lieutenant U.S. Marine Corps.

impending doom, and suffered for two days with diarrhea, as a result of nervous stress and the side effects of a fifth of whiskey. The poor man had been stationed at the hospital for more than a year, and in that time he had seen corpsmen that had worked with him receiving FMF orders. Within a few months they were back as casualties or had fallen in combat.

Lieutenant Senior Grade William Flood and I had been medical school classmates, fellow general practitioners in Vermont, and now had orders for the west coast. The Skipper cut our orders so that we could travel together. We did so in a 1950 Plymouth sedan and made it to San Francisco in 4-1/2 days. A Marine Corps lieutenant colonel contacted us and agreed to pay for the gasoline if we would take him with us. This was a mistake. There are not many bad Marine Corps officers. This guy was bad. He stayed drunk in the back seat, most of the time and complained about everything.

One day we stopped off in Amarillo, Texas. The evening was highlighted when a rancher, who was apparently very wealthy, treated us with a gourmet meal and drinks. He made many complimentary speeches. I guess they hadn't seen many men in uniform there since the second world war. Meantime, our lieutenant colonel had gone out and picked up a couple of girls. The next morning he insisted on bringing them in the car with us, which would have crossed a state border, and been in violation of the Mann Act. Bill and I got the girls aside and paid them some money and threatened them with violence if they didn't make a hasty retreat.

Once in San Francisco, Bill and I checked in to the Marine Memorial Hotel. Here we had a real taste of military "hurry up and wait". It would be at least a week before we could expect transportation to Japan and Bill was informed that his LST was still at sea headed in our direction.

Actually, we thoroughly enjoyed our week in San Francisco, especially after we found the Navy Officer's Club and its excellent food.

After two and a half weeks, I said goodbye to Bill and boarded a four engine propeller plane for Japan. This was quite exciting for me. I suspect, more so than the others aboard, for this was my first flight on a plane of this size. My previous experience had been limited to flying lessons in a Piper Cub and flying in small one engine planes.

The 42 hour trip from San Francisco to Japan went by rapidly. We stopped briefly at Honolulu and Wake Island. The plane landed at Heneda Airport on the outskirts of Tokyo in the early evening. I was driven directly to the building then occupied by the United States Navy, and reported to the Admiral's office.

"Welcome to Japan, Lieutenant," he didn't call me doctor. "I have orders transferring you to the Marine Corps. You will receive your orders at the general's office." I didn't say anything, but thought, this is the first time I have seen an admiral, now I am going to see a Marine Corps general, not bad for a country boy.

I made my way to Marine Headquarters without much difficulty and handed my orders to a major, sitting at the desk guarding the general's office. He read the orders and buzzed the general.

"The general will see you now, Lieutenant."

Much to my surprise, the general was a real fine gentleman. He immediately set me at ease and asked me to take a chair.

"Lieutenant, you are going to join the first Marine Division in Korea. They are in the northeast on the 38th parallel at the present time where it is rather cold. Did you have training at Pickle Meadows?" (Pickle Meadows is an area high in the mountains in California where the marines receive their cold weather training.)

"No sir," I answered, "but I grew up in the mountains of Vermont where it is quite cold in the wintertime."

We chatted briefly about our personal lives and then he told me that the major would cut orders for me for my transportation to southwestern Japan where, at Atami Airbase, I would take a flight to Pohang, which at the time had a code name and was a Marine Corps Airbase.

"Sir, how do I travel from Tokyo to Atami?"

"By train," he answered.

"I have no knowledge of the Japanese language. Do they speak English?" I asked.

"No, but you'll make out all right," he assured me.

"Sir, what do I do after I reach Pohang?"

"You will not receive orders here," he informed me, "but at Pohang you will take a twin engine plane over the mountains to Chun Chon and from there you will take a single engine observation plane to join the marines located in the punchbowl area." He then gave me my verbal assignment and very nicely outlined the details of my assignment before I again reported to the major.

By then it was 9 o'clock in the evening. The major was closing up shop and said,

"Come on, lieutenant, I'll buy you a drink." I needed some sleep, not a drink, but I guess there was no choice.

We went out onto the streets and I had my real first glimpse of the Oriental race. The full impact of my status as a foreigner hit me as this new race of people with their strange language, gait, honeybuckets, wooden shoes, and baby backpacks came into view. There were hundreds and hundreds of bicycles. The three-wheeled motor vehicles, stores, music, and the many activities making up the busy Japanese street scene opened up a new and different world for me. We had gone less than one block before some street walkers came up asking us in broken English if we wanted a girl for the evening, or night, at a real reasonable price.

The major and I went into a cabaret. It was the same thing over again. I wondered why there were so many prostitutes. They were poor. Nearly everyone was poor in Japan in the post World War II days.

I was trying to digest some of this while we were sipping our drinks. I guess I didn't say very much and the major most likely thought I was a bore or possibly he realized I was tired.

"Come on, Lieutenant, I have a place for you to sleep tonight," he said bringing me to a very clean, small Japanese hotel. He paid the person at the front desk and brought me to my room. "Here's some yen (money), Lieutenant. You may have a visitor during the night and will need this. You can pay me back tomorrow when we get you set for your little trip."

"What do you mean visitor?" I asked.

"You'll see," he answered as he departed.

I had just gotten to sleep when I heard the door sliding open. There had been no knock. I sat up in bed and wished I had a weapon. Soon I realized it was a very attractive young Japanese lady.

"You wanta me? Only three hundra yen." I didn't know it at the time, but this was less than one dollar. There were 360 yen for each American dollar at the time. She seemed a bit hurt when I told her no, but turned around and departed as quickly and silently as she had come.

The next morning I was up bright and early waiting in the lobby for the major. He appeared at 0730 and brought me back to headquarters where I was ill-fitted for a Marine Corps uniform with silver bars on each shoulder and shirt collar. They managed to fit all of my cold weather gear into one long, slender cylindrical duffel bag which was marked: "Wm. W. Montgomery, M.C., USMC 1st Marine Division, FMF FPO San Francisco, Calif." I still use this duffel bag.

I never saw the major again. A Marine Corps sergeant brought me to the train station in Tokyo. The train ride from Tokyo to Kyoto and then on to Atami took an entire day and a good portion of the evening. My train ride ended when I reached the station at Atami. Not a word of English had reached my ears the entire day. Feeling rather forlorned and deserted, I could hardly wait to get rid of my heavy pack and find a place to sleep. Stepping from the train, I followed the only English signs in the station area. These were marked RTO and led me to a small unheated shack. Inside the doorway was a drinking water container on my left and a chair on the right. The only other piece of furniture was a small desk and chair in the center of the room whose sole ornaments were a telephone and a Japanese railroad man. He rose and bowed. I slid my pack to the floor and awkwardly returned the gesture.

"Good evening. Can you tell me how I can get to the Marine Corps camp?" I asked.

"Intupita no heah. Me no speak," was his answer. I sat down in the chair. Half an hour passed and no interpreter appeared. The railroad man's eyes never left me. Occasionally he would smile. Another half hour passed. For the most part I avoided his stare, but my eyes did wander in the direction of the desk and then the telephone. The telephone! Why not try the telephone? I walked over to the desk, pointed to the telephone, and then into my mouth, and looked him straight in the eyes. He nodded his head up and down, so I picked up the phone.

"Hello? Mushi. Mushi." (Someone had told me to say "mushi, mushi" when talking on the telephone.)

"Halo."

"Do you speak English?"

"Yas."

"Please ring Marine Corps." He contacted a third party, talked in Japanese a few seconds and then everything went silent. I rang the operator again, repeated my request and ended with the same degree of success. Since it was no colder outside, and the stare of my companion was becoming rather annoying, I picked up my gear and walked out into the street. An hour later I spotted a Marine Corps jeep and waved him down. This became my transportation to the marine base.

I checked into the BOQ (Bachelor Officer's Quarters). After unpacking my toilet gear, I proceeded down to the shower room for a much needed cleansing. Soon, two women appeared in the shower room with me. They were obviously cleaning ladies, "Come on, get out of here! Can't you see I'm taking a shower?" I shouted rather startled,

"No problem sir," they replied, but continued to clean and did not leave. This was my introduction to the fact that there was no room for modesty in the Orient!

The flight from Atami, Japan to Pohang, Korea the next day was uneventful. The temperature in Pohang had dropped sufficiently so that it was necessary for me to put on my winter gear.

"God, if it's this cold in southeastern Korea, what's it going to be like in the mountains up in the north?" I was soon to find out.

The Marine Air Corps officer's club at Pohang Dong was a very pleasant surprise. Typical of pilots, they had a tent converted into a regular saloon, except that there were no women. I spent a very pleasant evening talking with the pilots. They flew heavy propellered bombers and saber jets. One of the pilots was a famous Red Sox baseball player. This was my last taste of civilized living for some time.

Several other marines traveled with me from Pohang up to Chun Chon in a twin engine plane. From here I hopped a single engine scout plane for my final destination. As we traveled over the mountains of higher elevation, the turbulence became worse and worse. If I had not had experience in a single engine plane earlier on in life, I am sure I would have been airsick. We didn't talk much.

Finally, just before we reached our destination, the sergeant flying the plane said, "Lieutenant, I would appreciate it if you would get all ready to jump out when we land. Up here I'm a sitting duck for a sniper and I certainly don't want to run into a machine gun." A nice guy. What about me? I didn't answer him. My stomach began to rumble a bit and I expected a little action at either end of my intestinal tract at any moment. Fortunately none occurred and I felt better after I had jumped from the plane and was under cover away from the clearing where we landed.

Man, was it cold! I got out my map, checked where I was and then located a Marine Corps installation. It was not difficult to locate. A Corporal led me to a tent which was warmed by a potbellied stove. Thus began my adventure with warfare in a frigid zone. Soon I had a wealth of knowledge about clothing, living conditions, food, weapon handling and the like, and also a very good idea as to the exact location of outfits in most sectors along the front. My mission was to obtain confidential information, which was never any problem because I was wearing the uniform of a United States Marine.

I checked out a 45 automatic pistol, a weapon that was to be my constant companion during my entire stay in combat. It was a new gun but the holster was somewhat used. At this point I certainly was thankful for my having had training in its handling and field stripping. I had also become a fair shot with the 45 automatic and a carbine automatic rifle.

The response of the body as it is introduced to a frigid zone is of interest to a medical person. When entering a frigid zone, such as North Korea in the winter, the adjustment of the body to the cold is an automatic physiological function. This, of course, must be assisted by the proper use of clothing and shelter. The exposure to cold climate causes the blood vessels to constrict. This produces a cooler skin and thus decreases sweating, thereby conserving body heat. The thyroid gland becomes more active and its increased secretion of thyroxine causes the body to increase its output of heat. The heat center in the brain becomes acclimated to cold weather and decreases the sensitivity to cold stimulus. Personnel arriving in the cold weather zone during the summer or fall can easily adjust to the gradually increasing cold. This adjustment is much more difficult for troops arriving in the winter. It is for this reason that the military forces have set up a cold weather training camp in the mountains of California. I had my training in the hills of Vermont.

In order to lighten my pack, and also to keep warm, I had worn many layers of clothing, including a set of woolen underwear, heavy pants, wind proof pants, a woolen shirt, sweater, parka, two pairs of socks and rubber insulated boots. Over all of this I wore a woolen coat and, of course, a woolen hat under my helmet.

The next day I stood around in the cold and snow until late afternoon waiting for a convoy to form which would be headed in the direction of the "punchbowl". At about 4 o'clock we departed from the region of the airstrip in 4x4 trucks. We rode on fairly smooth dirt roads near the seashore for half an hour and then the trucks began to climb the mountains. When the sun set the temperature dropped well below zero. The bumps on the road were unmerciful and without letup. We passed through many war torn villages with only the remnants of shacks remaining by the sides of the road. Women and children streamed from these huts as we approached and begged for food as we passed. A few candy bars were tossed here and there. On several occasions, I attempted to converse with the marine on either side of me as we were seated on benches on both sides of the truck.

"How long is this going to take?" I asked.

No answer. He obviously could not hear me. I yelled over the noise of the truck and he turned to me.

"I don't know, but I wish we would get somewhere. My ass is killing me and I've got to take another leak!" Further conversation was just too much effort - noise, bumps, cold, dust.

Two hours passed. The convoy stopped. On one side of the road was a straight walled cliff rising at least 75 feet. On the other side was an abrupt drop to a gully 50 feet below. Everyone hobbled from the trucks to perform the long overdue necessities. We limbered our aching backs and attempted to remove some of the caked dust from our noses. The dust in Korea during the winter months is nearly as bad as it is during the summer. This dust is very fine and penetrates every pore of the skin, forming a rooted base for additional layers. Dressed as I was, I later found layers of this dust, as thick as they were on my face, in my axilla and groin regions. This would not be removed for many months.

As we were standing there in the road we heard a sound as though something were churning or chopping the air. As this sound became more audible, a large helicopter came into view.

"Ah, I thought, this is modern warfare. They are bringing us hot coffee and food." Ha! I had a lot to learn. The convoy had radioed ahead for gasoline.

We arrived at Division Headquarters at 9 p.m. that evening. It seemed like a 12 hour trip but had only been 5 hours. Once there, I wished we were back on the truck, or better still, back in the USA. The sound of incoming and outgoing artillery fire on the MLR (maximum line of resistance) was frightening. I didn't say anything. I was a bit scared and I'm sure those who had been there a while saw me coming and knew it.

After a few days it wasn't so bad. It is amazing how soon one compensates for this increase in environmental noise. It becomes part of everyday activity and is somehow mentally subdued. I imagine this is similar to a city dweller becoming adjusted to traffic noise. There is, however, one difference. When incoming shells are getting closer and closer, and you feel yourself becoming part of the target, an almost instant alarm system sends you in search of a bunker or foxhole.

"Damn, I wish I had something to eat and drink!" I looked at the snow and thought about eating it as I did when I was a kid. By this time, my pack was getting mighty heavy. Mostly I was cold. It had to be well below zero. I found a rather large tent with a sign over the entrance "Division Headquarters". I banged on the door one time, opened it, walked in and dropped my pack. The occupants were two marine lieutenants who were sitting at a desk made from crating lumber. A pot bellied stove was red with heat and the tent was warm. A couple of cots with sleeping bags on them were in the corner of the tent and were the only other furnishings. I introduced myself and announced that I would like to talk with the Division Surgeon. One of the officers was a second lieutenant, the other a first lieutenant. The first lieutenant asked me for my orders.

"I have verbal orders to report directly to the Division Surgeon."

"You gotta have written orders to get anywhere up here, Doc," he informed me. Now, just in case I ran into a Bozo like this I did have a slip of paper folded up and concealed in the inside pocket of my field jacket which was signed by the commandant in Tokyo. These orders read For the Investigation of Medical Matters

"Just what do these orders mean, Doc?"

"Just what is says, lieutenant. I am to report to the Division Surgeon for a discussion of medical matters."

The door opened and several other officers reported in for duty. I stepped aside and sat on my pack. After they departed, both lieutenants all of a sudden became real friendly. I think the lack of information must have aroused their curiosity. They knew I was a doctor for they spotted the cadeusus on my collar opposite the collar with the silver bars.

"Doc, the Division Surgeon is away for a day or two. Why don't you bunk in here with us? We'll call for an additional cot and sleeping bag.

At least it's warm."

They both asked me several more questions concerning military matters, got no answers, and then started chatting about personal matters and asked me how things were back in the States.

"You guys got anything to eat?" I asked.

"Sure, we're just about to put together some chow."

The second lieutenant pulled a few cans from a cardboard carton and a Coleman burner which had been stored under his cot. He lit the burner and soon I had my first taste of coffee in the field. This, along with some K-rations and cookies, was a real treat. I was hungry.

At about noon the next day, I was introduced to the Division Surgeon. I discussed with him the nature of my mission and that I was to work as a Medical Officer at the MASH level, when not pursuing my activity of interrogation. He signed a small pass for me which gave me access to all areas on the front.

The following morning I set out in the direction of the front line, which was referred to as the punchbowl. My transportation was a jeep, my driver a marine corporal. As we neared the front line, the increasing volume of the noise of warfare was both exciting and rather sickening. It was exciting because of the danger and the novelty. I was now a part of an active war, something I had frequently daydreamed about most of my life, as I am sure other boys do. What would it be like to see the front line where men fight and die? I was now to find out. The sickening sensation stemmed from the thought that as I listened to the sound of guns, there were men in pain and men dying.

My investigation led me from the front lines back to the hospital ship off the southeastern coast of Korea. Thus, I had ample opportunity to study many of the aspects of cold weather evacuation of casualties as well as the living conditions in the frigid zone. It might be of interest even to layman, to learn of the evacuation techniques in frigid zone warfare. I will accomplish this by discussing the immediate therapy of the wounded followed by the various techniques of evacuation.

The corpsman is usually the first person to reach the wounded. He must, after dragging or carrying them to cover and away from direct fire, consider the degree of shock. Shock follows most war injuries. A degree of shock can accompany even a minor wound because of the psychological, or so-called vagal-vagal (fainting) response of the body. There is a slowing down of the circulatory system and the skin becomes cold and clammy. Then, he may suffer from air hunger and may vomit, or may pass into an unconscious state. Shock is our first consideration in war injuries, just as it is in those injuries that occur in civilian life. A good corpsman probably has more to do with the prevention and treatment of shock than does the doctor, for the initial treatment is of utmost importance. This is especially true in cold weather warfare. What does a corpsman do to prevent or restore the collapse of body function? First, he must look for bleeding. Quite often hemorrhage can be controlled by the application of a battle dressing. If the dressing does not suffice, he must apply pressure or a tourniquet. The time and application of a tourniquet is recorded on the evacuation tag which the corpsman carries on the inside pocket of his field jacket. In cold weather the tourniquet should be loosened every 15-20 minutes.

Warmth is the corpsman's next consideration. When under fire and treating a wounded marine, he usually does not have access to rapid evacuation. In a frigid zone, getting the wounded marine into a sleeping bag would be ideal. The corpsman may sacrifice his own jacket. I knew more than one corpsman who suffered frostbite as a result of this sacrifice. We had available chemical heating pads to which about an ounce of water was added. This, placed in a sleeping bag along with the patient, provided warmth and comfort. Before being wounded, the marine is usually quite active and now he is suddenly inactive. The circulation is depressed and his production of body heat is decreased. He may be quite wet from bleeding, and if this increases the heat loss, the wounded soldier is in imminent danger of either freezing or entering irreversible shock.

As soon as the bleeding is under control and all available measures have been taken to keep the patient warm, the corpsman must consider pain. Pain is controlled by the injection of morphine tartrate from a syrette. These syrettes look like tiny toothpaste tubes with a needle on one end. The corpsmen and Battalion Surgeons carry these syrettes of morphine next to the body to prevent them from freezing. The time and dose of morphine is recorded on the patient's evacuation tag. If the initial dose of morphine is not recorded and the pain is not relieved because of delayed absorption into the bloodstream (a result of the cold and shock), the casualty may receive repeated injections of morphine as he is evacuated in the direction of an Aid Station. When he finally does reach this Aid Station, or Medical Company, where he is warmed and further treated for shock, the absorption of morphine from the injection sites into the bloodstream suddenly becomes apparent by symptoms of overdose or even death. It is thus imperative that each injection of morphine be recorded on the casualty's evacuation tag. Most often the corpsman will have a supply of serum albumin. An intravenous infusion of serum albumin is imperative if the patient has had much bleeding or is in shock.

Fractures must be immobilized before the casualty is moved. Usually the corpsman does not have splints and he must improvise. When nothing else is available, a fractured arm can be fixed to the body or a fractured leg can be strapped to and splinted by the other leg.

When the corpsman finishes his initial first aid treatment, he must then consider evacuation. This is pretty well organized for the corpsman during large operations. All casualties are carried to the forward Aid Station directly behind the battle. A forward Aid Station is composed of one or two doctors, several corpsmen, a vast amount of medical supplies, three or four field ambulances and one to three of the bell-type helicopters ("whirlybirds") that can evacuate two casualties during one flight.

The doctor performs emergency treatments and supervises the evacuations. The latter function requires a considerable amount of skill and discretion. Routes of evacuation must not be overcrowded and care must be taken to make sure that the proper casualties are evacuated by helicopter.

The corpsman has the sole responsibility for the management of a casualty when he is on a small operation such as a scouting patrol. The advice of the battalion doctor is not available unless there are radio communications from the patrol to the battalion headquarters. If he is unable to stop the bleeding or control the process of shock, his best bet is to stay put in a safe place and send a runner back for a helicopter evacuation, or instruct the field phone operator to call for one. Helicopters as a rule are not supposed to go beyond the front line and into enemy territory. Fortunately, the Marine pilots did not adhere to this regulation in the case of real emergencies.

Carrying a casualty back to the line and away from enemy fire is no easy task in the summer. Think of what it must be like with a couple of feet of snow, subzero temperatures and a piercing wind. Manipulation of a hand litter in the snow covered terrain is next to impossible. A litter attached to a toboggan is the most practical means of evacuating a casualty in the snow. After reaching the rear, the casualty is transferred to a jeep or field ambulance, provided there is one available, and if there is a road. The "weasel" is ideal for evacuating casualties in the snow. This is the same type of snow tractor that is seen in many ski resorts today.

As a general rule, if the casualty makes it to the battalion or regimental area, he "has it made", for he is only a short distance from a warm Janesway tent with two doctors, a number of corpsmen, and excellent surgical facilities to care for him.

If at all possible, seriously wounded casualties are evacuated directly to a medical company (MASH) by helicopter. The casualties are placed in the litter capsules attached on each side of the helicopters landing gear. These capsules are warmed from the helicopters engines and it is a matter of minutes before they reach the medical company. It was a real boost to the morale of the fighting troops to know that they could be evacuated in a matter of minutes, safely and comfortably, to a medical company which is equipped with the best of modern medical gear.

Minor wounds were evacuated from the battalion level to the regimental sick bay tent. Casualties not serious enough to be evacuated by helicopter, but too severe to be treated at the regimental level, are evacuated directly to the medical company by jeep or field ambulance. This is not a comfortable ride.

Occasionally, the management of casualties was not as well organized as I have outlined above. This is especially true when following the marines during a "push" or forward advance. There, of course, were no tents, and we would dig foxholes before or as the battle began. We carried with us our medical and surgical supplies which included a large number of bottles of serum albumin and plasma. They would carry the casualties back to us with everything from a litter to an armored tank. We had equipment to perform emergency operations such as a tracheotomy, or suturing of blood vessels on the loose. During these times we worked our butts off, often for two or three days without sleep. I guess our main job was to sort the wounded. The dead were placed to one side, the critically injured evacuated by helicopter, and the rest by jeep or field ambulance. When there were large numbers, they were piled into trucks. Think about what a ride that must have been. The medical company in the Marine Corps (MASH) is composed of from 8 to 15 doctors, a large team of corpsmen, and a relatively small group of marines. There were no nurses. A casualty arriving at the Medical Company is carried into a large rectangular squad tent, and placed in his stretcher onto rails which run the length of the tent. These rails are about three feet in height and eight feet apart. This area in the squad tent is known as the receiving room. Here, wounds are examined and redressed. Whole blood is first available at this level. We used type O positive blood, which is the universal donor type. We did not type and cross-match before administering

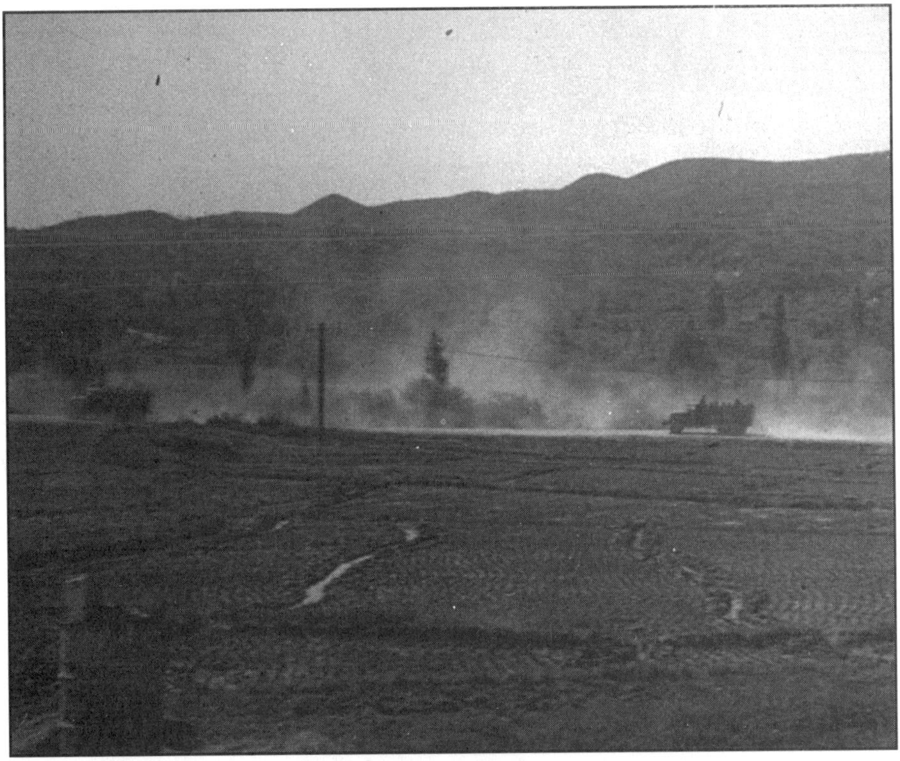

Dust and more dust. It was impossible to keep clean when on the move.

the blood, sort of a Russian Roulette as far as reactions are concerned. The receiving tent is equipped with a portable X-ray unit for the localization of missiles and shrapnel as well as the evaluation of fractures.

If the wounds are not severe, the casualty is carried to an adjacent and connected squad tent, known as the debridement, minor surgical tent. Here the minor wounds are excised and as much shrapnel removed as is possible or practical. The wounds are then approximated using wire suture material. Catgut suture is used to ligate bleeding blood vessels.

More serious cases are carried to another squad tent, with railing similar to those in the receiving room. Here they await surgery. Connected to this squad tent is a double Janesway, which is an insulated tent in the shape of a quonset hut and has a wooden floor. The double Janesway tent is just large enough for two operating tables head to head. The doctors administering anesthesia sit out of the way and in between the two operating tables. Usually the operating instruments and other equipment are sterilized at a point more distant from the front lines. Some medical companies have their own sterilizing setups.

After the casualties have recovered sufficiently (usually a few days) from their initial surgery at the medical company, they are transported to the hospital ship using field ambulances and liberty boats. Surgical cases requiring immediate specialized surgery are flown to the hospital ship from the medical company as soon as they are treated for shock. The larger helicopters with inborn litters were used for this type of transportation.

The greatest advance in the evacuation of casualties during the Korean War was the helicopter. Mr. Igor Sikorsky had every reason to be proud of his more than 30 years of tedious labor in the development of his wonderful "whirlybird".

All casualties occurring in winter warfare are by no means due to war wounds. During the first two winters of the Korean War, a very large number of Marines were evacuated suffering from frostbite, immersion foot, or trench foot. Trench foot applies to cold injuries affecting the feet of soldiers who stood for long periods in cold and damps foxholes and trenches. Frostbite is a cold injury not necessarily associated with dampness. Immersion foot originally was a nautical term applied to a syndrome resulting from immersion of the feet in cold sea water, such as in a life raft for a long period of time. Frostbite is most common in the nose, face, ears, hands and feet. The first sensation is that of pain and then numbness. If the feet are involved, the victim is noted to have a clumsy gait. The feet at this time are swollen, pale, and insensitive to touch. The arterial pulsations to the foot are absent. In a few days, the part affected by frostbite becomes red, swollen, hot and dry. The pulse is returned and accentuated. Large blisters and blebs appear. Instead of a numbness, the part becomes hypersensitive even to the lightest touch. There is a continuous burning sensation. This stage can last for over two weeks, then if the cold injury has been severe, the part becomes black. This is the picture of dry gangrene. The part may become infected resulting in cellulitis or "blood poisoning". If the injury has not been severe enough to progress through gangrene, there still may be some permanent damage to the blood vessels, and a hypersensitivity to cold and pain with exercise may persist for the rest of the casualty's life. Also, the affected part is very prone to repeat frostbite even with a minimal exposure to cold. We had a few "don'ts" for the immediate treatment of cold injury. The affected parts were not to be rubbed. Snow should not be applied. Rapid warming, such as in warm water, is very harmful. All marines receive instruction as to the treatment of cold injuries, otherwise these "don'ts" would most certainly not be carried out.

The most important consideration during frigid weather warfare other than fighting equipment, is the soldier's clothing. In many instances there was no shelter or means of heat. Clothing was the sole defense against the cold. Underwear consisting of 50% wool and cotton fabric is best for general use. Tight clothing decreases the circulation in the extremities. Excessive clothing can cause perspiration, a dampening of the fabric, and then an increased danger for cold injury. The introduction of windproof, water-repellent pants and jackets greatly improved the comfort of the fighting men in frigid zones. This cloth, in addition to being windproof and water-repellent, must not be sufficiently airtight as to prevent the transmission of insensible perspiration.

The marines in Korea were the first to use the so-called "thermo-boots" in combat. This boot was designed to employ the vapor barrier principle which consists of a layer of synthetic wool covered inside and out by a layer of rubber. This boot is far superior to the Shoepak, Mukluk, and Felt boot. The thermo-boot is, however, not foolproof and must be used properly to control excessive sweating and maceration of the skin. The boot should be not too tight around the leg so that it can "breathe" and prevent excessive sweating. "Athlete's foot" thrives in a warm, damp environment. Anhydrotic "antisweating" footpowder is used whenever possible. Socks should be changed twice in any 24 hour period. An extra pair of socks is dried over a stove, in a sleeping bag, or next to the body. The feet should be thoroughly dried and lightly massaged at the time of changing socks. As the Marines in Korea became accustomed to the proper usage of the thermo-boot, the incidence of cold injury to the feet reduced markedly.

I found the service handgear to be quite inadequate to keep my hands warm and was most grateful to have brought a pair of ski mittens with me. I wore these over heavy woolen mittens. Metal and ice should not be touched by the bare hands in subzero temperatures, for the skin will become firmly adherent. When this occurred, many became panicky and during the process of pulling away, lost a bit of skin. This incident occurs quite commonly in winter warfare for everyone carries a weapon which is difficult to handle when wearing heavy gloves or mittens. When it does occur, there is only one thing to do. Pee on it.

When the temperature dropped below 10 or 20 below zero, it was difficult to keep warm, especially at night. Winter sleeping bags were made of an outer windresistant, water-repellent fabric and an inner nylon lining. Between these two layers was a quilted layer of down. Since sleeping bags were quite plentiful, many had two bags, one inside the other. Sleeping with your face inside a sleeping bag or in damp sweaty clothes, was an invitation to a sleepless night. At one time I found a couple of hand warmers and placed these inside the sleeping bag during subzero weather. One of these warmers, filled with cigarette lighter fluid, lasted at least 12 hours. After you got used to the smell, these little buggers made a difference between a good night's sleep and a night of tossing and turning.

One cold day, while I was out in a blinding snowstorm in Korea, I flashed back to my childhood, walking up Barns Street on my way to school in Vermont during a blizzard. I don't ever remember their closing school during a snow storm. It was less than a mile's walk for me, but more than two miles for many of the other kids. We walked it and loved it. It was great growing up in a small Vermont town!

As I think back, there is a strong possibility that I may have frozen to death if I had not grown up in the mountains of Vermont and knew how to cope with living outdoors in 20 below zero weather.

At the time I joined the first Marine Division, they had recently retreated from the "Frozen Choshin" reservoir region and were back in the vicinity of the 38th parallel, on the east coast in the mountains. This area was called the "Punchbowl".

The fighting at this time was not very intense, for the enemy had backed up a ways. In addition to occasional bursts from artillery shells or mortars, we were always on the lookout for snipers and infiltrators who accounted for a fair number of casualties with their burp gun bullets and grenades. It's pretty much a statement of fact, that nocturnal fear far exceeds that during the day. Often at night I would stay awake looking up at the hole which had been constructed in the roof of the bunker to allow smoke to escape, or to house a stove pipe which was connected to a potbellied stove. If an infiltrator dropped a grenade into one of these it was "certain curtains".

I'd been a long way and seen an almost incomprehensible number of new things, so foreign to my existence as a general practitioner in a small Vermont town. There were so many new things to look at, new wounds to hear and new odors, most pleasant, some foreign and unpleasant. In some ways, to a country boy, this was almost like being on a different planet. I could feel, or sense, this new environment. Yet I was the same person. I felt the same as I did back in Vermont. It certainly made a tremendous impression on me, but thus far there were no dents. I often thought about this, for it was quite obvious that many of the medical personnel attached to the Marines in combat were somewhat devastated by their new existence. Was I stupid or insensitive? I finally concluded that even though being in combat was stressful, it was no more so than the day to day life of a busy general practitioner in a small country town, with long hours of hard work, stress, and a constant lack of sleep - except for the sporadic attacks of fear with the thoughts of being wounded or killed.

Chapter Fifteen

FIELD MEDICINE

In the spring of 1952, The First Marine Division moved from the freezing winter front in the mountains on the eastern coast of Korea to the warmer summer front on the western coast. The heavy fighting had suddenly shifted from east to west and "where the going gets tough, the marines get going." I was convinced that the United States Marine Corps was the most spirited, the best trained and well-disciplined military organization in the world, and I was proud to be with them.

While I was in Seoul, waiting for the truck convoy that would take us to the front, a marine line officer offered to take me on a jeep tour of the city. Poverty and despair were everywhere. It seemed that the people who had money were the Koreans working for the military forces, the black marketeers or the numerous prostitutes. The rest of the Korean population was hungry.

Prostitution, by far, was the biggest business, followed by the black marketeering. It was only a small percentage of people who worked for the military doing manual labor, or being houseboys for some of the officers at the regimental and division levels. I was impressed that these people were quiet, polite, strong and hard working. It was difficult to determine the degree of their intelligence, for I only understood a few words of the Korean language and most of them didn't speak English or Japanese.

The North and South Korean Armies and the United States Marine Force had accomplished a thorough debridement of the war-torn Seoul. The only structure I saw untouched was the Capitol building. It was explained to me that when the North Korean Army occupied Seoul, they had used the Capitol building as a horse stable to insult the South Koreans. There was, as yet, no sign of reconstruction. This, of course, was out of the question with another siege of the city still within reach of the plausible.

I left Seoul, and a five hour truck ride brought me to the MLR, and again the sound of artillery, rockets, mortars and small arms fire echoed in the air and became a part of my life.

During the lull in 1951, when the Peace Talks began, each side had ample opportunity to strengthen its lines. When fighting resumed, advancement was impossible, for the most impregnable lines were supplemented with the high mountains on the east coast.

The United Nation Forces had better equipment and better trained fighting men. Our fighting tactics consisted of using long range bombing and close air support. The Chinese and the North Koreans didn't have these capabilities. With this military superiority, we should have advanced easily, but we didn't. The reason seemed to be the endless supply of Communist manpower the enemy had at their disposal. During some of the larger battles, I am sure the better part of many of the Chinese regiments were destroyed, but before the United Nation Forces could be organized to push further north, or even hold the advancement, another Chinese regiment would be thrown into battle to replace the one that had been lost. In the end the result was a large number of human casualties and no gain or loss of territory by either side. The North Korean Communist offenses were, for the most part, completely fruitless against our artillery, rockets and close air support. We were told a number of times that there was some sort of deal between the two sides where if we didn't bomb north of the Yalub River, the Communists would not employ close air support and strafing. I firmly believed this was true.

The temperature was often 20 below zero in the winter and in the summer, days above 120 degrees Fahrenheit were common. I often think about which was worse and invariably come to the conclusion that it is a little better to be too hot than too cold. In the winter when it is real cold, you are conscious of it every minute of the day and night. It was impossible for me to sleep in an environment twenty degrees below zero. There is a much better chance of surviving if you are wounded when it is too hot vs. too cold. There is almost no way you can bathe when it is twenty below zero. Sometimes we went several months without a bath. Being raunchy is a real form of misery. It's the cold hands and feet that really get to you. They become stiff and it is a real effort to perform simple tasks such as unzipping or unbuttoning an article of clothing. It seemed like seconds before a cup of coffee or hot soup became cold in a tin cup. Cold makes your eyes water and your nose run. Tears freeze adding to your discomfort.

When it is hot, there are bugs...and snakes...and leeches...and you sweat. It is impossible to sleep without mosquito netting. Some of the guys had trouble sleeping when it was very hot. I never did, as long as I wasn't being bitten by bugs. There are more rats in the summer. When it is hot, food spoils quickly and the incidence of gastrointestinal infections increases. Everyone had intestinal worms. Malaria and other tropical diseases are prevalent, especially Manchurian fever, which was usually fatal.

Urinating in the summer was no problem. In the winter when it was very cold, if you happened to get some moisture on your zipper, and this gets fixed to the skin, it was very painful. Defecating in the wintertime is a major production, and constipation is a common entity among the troops. It is a real struggle all the way down to the long underwear. I won't go into detail, but it is quite a chore. It is not as bad in the summertime except that in order to keep any form of sanitation, holes must be dug. The odor from these is quite offensive. You can always count on more than two or three mosquito bites on your rear end. Otherwise, it's not so bad unless you get hit by a sniper bullet.

In the wintertime it is impossible to have any hobbies, other than blowing spit bubbles and the like. You can read, but it is very difficult to turn the pages. In the summertime when in the shade or in a tent, I could play cards or wood carve. The days were longer and reading was a real pleasure if you could find something to read. Once in a while we would

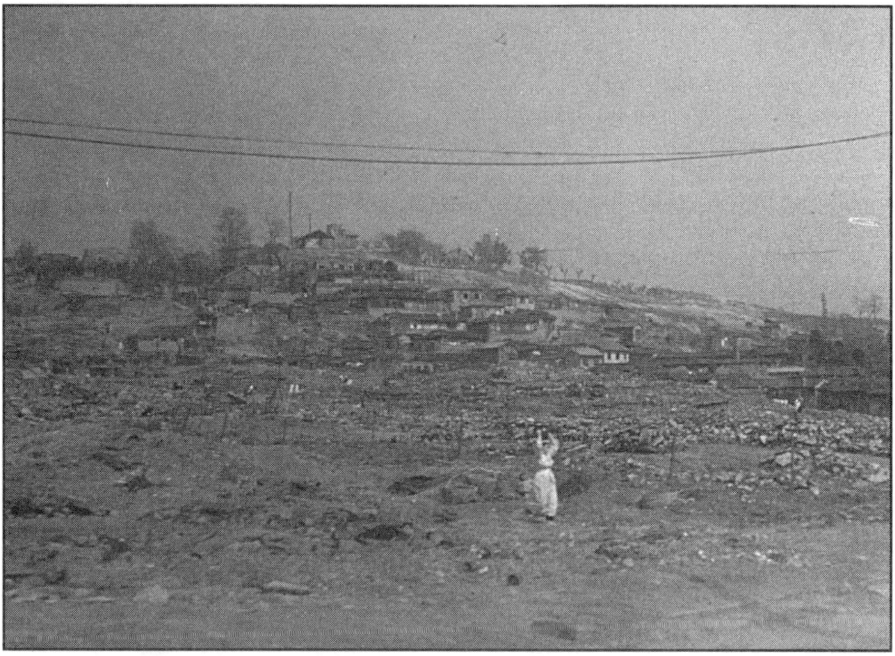

Seoul, Korea. Not much left after being besieged by both sides.

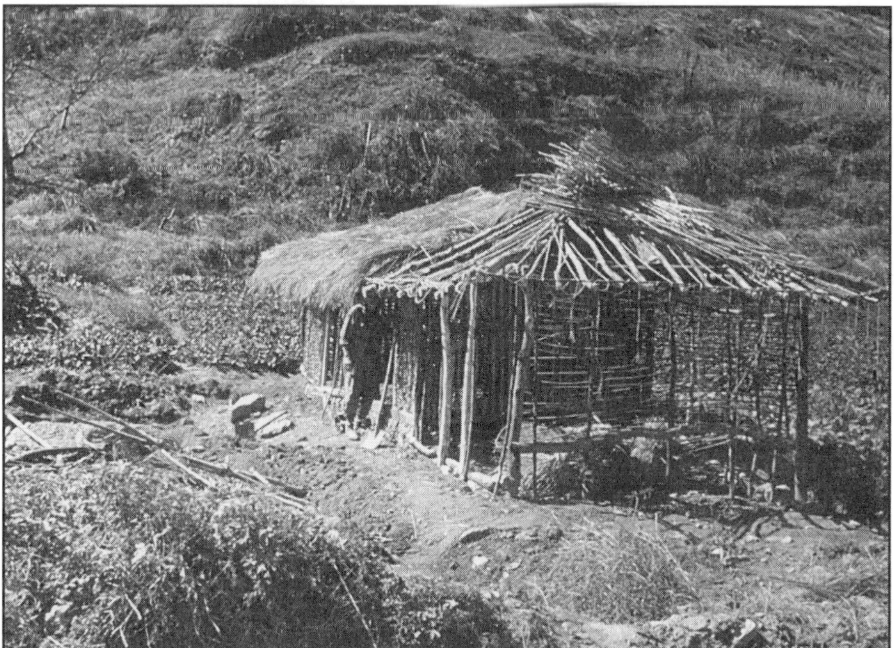

A farmer trying to rebuild.

have a volleyball game.

Driving a vehicle had its problems both in the winter and the summer. In the wintertime, it was difficult to start any vehicle. When they were running for a while, the heat from the vehicle was an absolute delight. Basically, the roads were smoother in the wintertime because of the snow, but there was the problem of frequently becoming stuck in the snow. In the summertime, the roads were in terrible condition due to frequent downpours. The potholes were everywhere. Often, you would encounter a small lake which had replaced the road after a thunderstorm. Military vehicles are not built for comfort. After many miles of bouncing up and down in the potholes, almost everyone would have a backache. Then it would dry out and the dust was almost unbearable, especially if we were traveling in a convoy.

The Chinese and North Koreans were great diggers. Both in the winter and summer, they lived underground when they were not fighting. As a general rule, there was a lull in fighting when it was very cold or very warm, but you couldn't count on it.

What was the Korean War like anyway, from the eyes of a medical officer? What did a medical officer do with his time other than treat the wounded? Many things - some of us even helped gather information

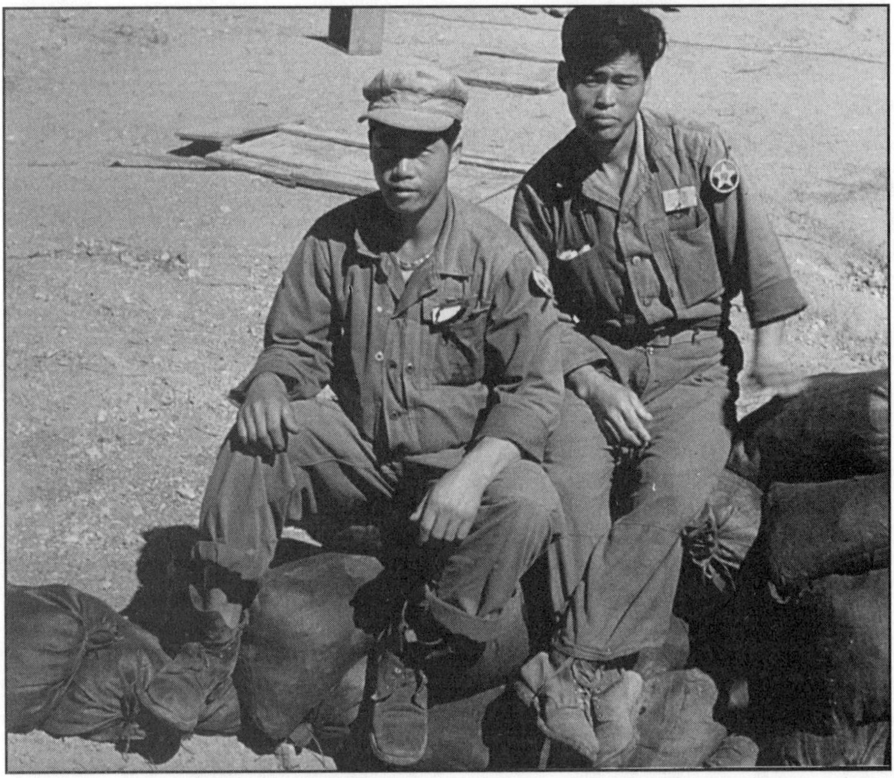

Two Korean service corps workers.

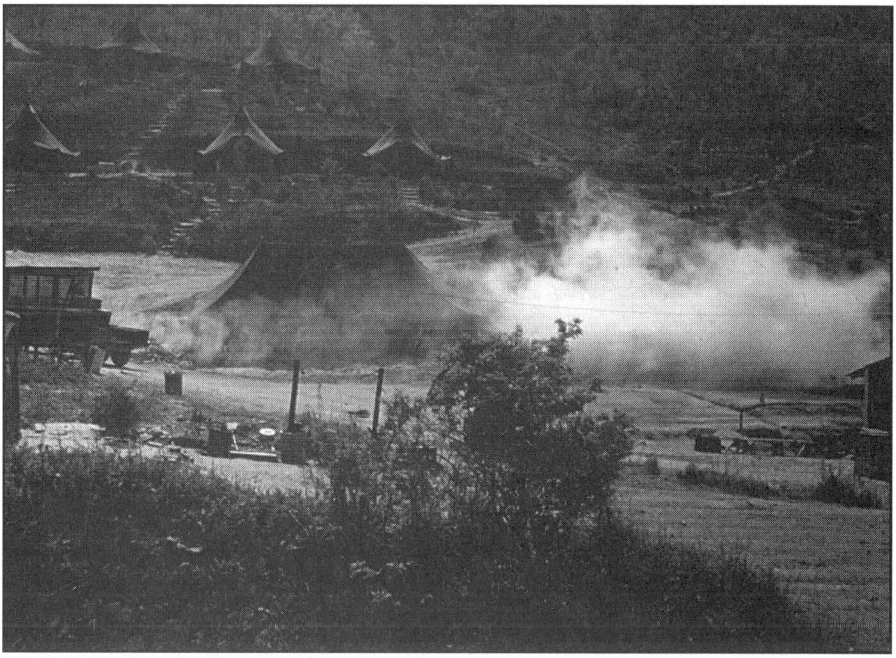

The mosquito population was controlled using a DDT spray. This photograph was taken back at the regimental level.

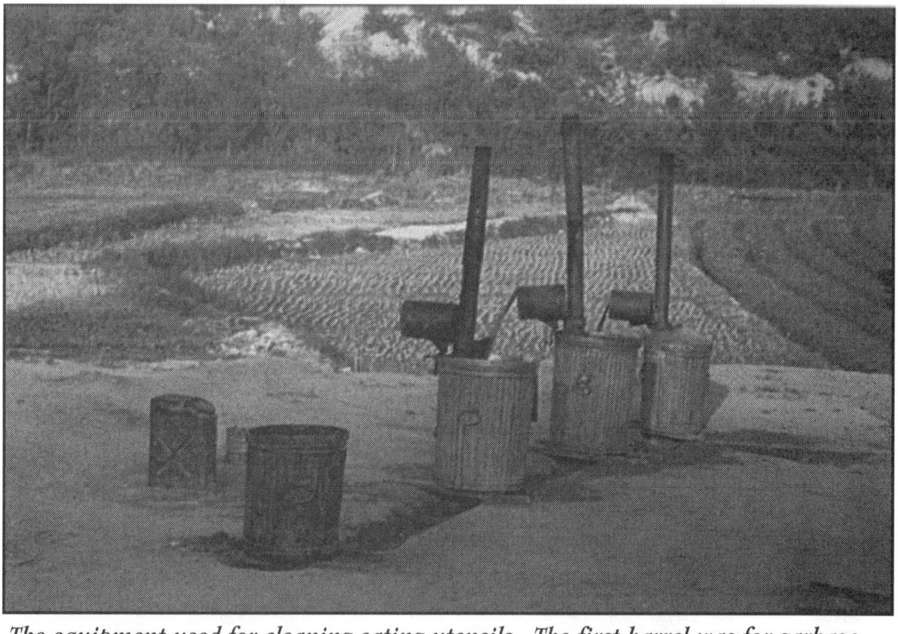

The equipment used for cleaning eating utensils. The first barrel was for garbage, the next barrel with the emersion burner was for washing utensils, and the other two are for rinsing in boiling water not less than 20 seconds.

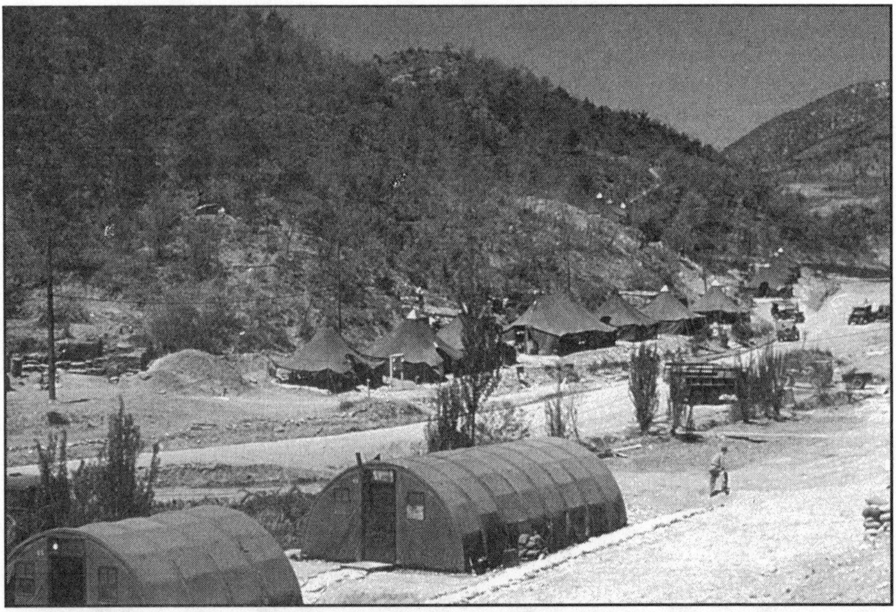

An area for the reserve battalion which is located approximately one mile behind the front line.

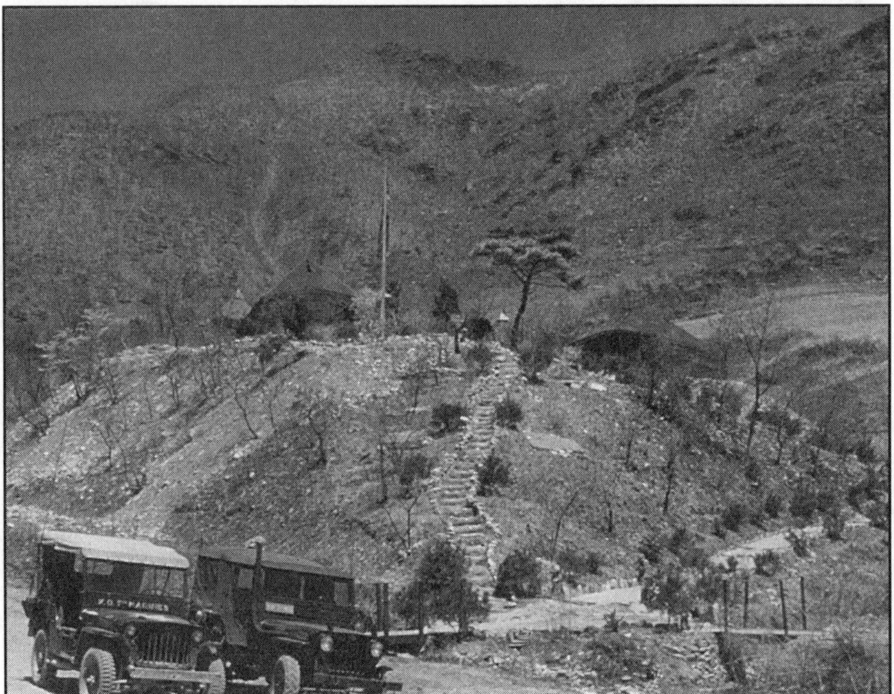

A view of the Colonel's living quarters at the Division Level.

from the enemy. Most of our duties, however, were grouped under the heading of "field sanitation".

"The medical officer must make inspections and recommendations to ensure the quality and nutritional adequacy of the rations." The prevention of food poisoning is a must at the front line. Such an epidemic could be worse than a large number of casualties. Can you imagine the marines fighting and at the same time coping with vomiting and diahhrea? My theory was that a good mess sergeant is the best preventive measure against food poisoning, as well as maintaining proper nutrition of the marines. It is the close supervision by the mess sergeant, rather than the periodic inspections by officers, that makes the difference between a hazardous and a well-operated mess. It is the duty of the doctor to inspect all aspects of the mess.

We used what are know as immersion oil burners, placed in large metal barrels, to heat the water for washing and rinsing food utensils. Each marine was required to follow closely a routine of a rinse, a good washing of his utensils in soap and hot water, followed by a rinsing in boiling water of not less than 20 seconds each. There were thus three barrels with immersion oil burners in a row to accomplish this.

Insect control was never entirely effective, but we tried. Whenever possible, the galley and food storage bunkers were screened. The food handlers, as well as the unprepared food, were inspected at frequent intervals. Flies have a way of getting into food and laying their eggs. Maggots are not an uncommon finding when you are living out of doors in a warm climate. On the MLR, the problem of food preparation was eliminated, for the marines on the front line live on rations obtained from cans. I still carry one of those little gadgets we used to open up the ration cans. We all had favorites. Mine were ham chunks and any kind of canned fruit.

The quality of food at all levels in Korea, I am sure, was unsurpassed by any military campaign to date in history. It's hard to believe, but during the hot summer months, even the men on the lines were supplied with ice cream on occasion. It was carried to them in insulated back packs. You can't imagine how good this tasted.

"The medical officer must locate sources of water and supervise its treatment for purification". When troops are on the move, water is purified by its being treated in the canteen with tincture of iodine or Halzone tablets. This water is by no means tasty, but it is safe. The so-called Lister bag is ideal for a campsite supply of drinking water. The Lister bag is a waterproof canvas container that has four faucets at its base. It is about 4 feet in height and 3 feet in diameter. Half a gram of hypochlorite (lye) is dissolved in a canteen of water and poured into the Lister bag. The bag is then filled with water and stirred with a clean stick. Each faucet is opened for a second or two. The bag is then ready for use. This device was a source of wonderment to me. Water remained quite cool even in very hot weather in a Lister bag, if it is hung in the shade of a tree. When a camp is established, an adequate supply of water can be maintained by periodic runs with water trailers. Hypochlorite is also added to this water for purification.

During the summer months, the corpsmen and I did most of our bathing in the river. If time permitted, we enjoyed a pleasant sunning while floating on our air mattresses. One day in July, 1952, when things were quiet, we tried our luck at fishing in the river with improvised equipment, and minnows. Either the equipment was inadequate or the fish were not biting, for when we started back to our campsite, we had only one fish, which resembled a channel catfish, and a half a can of minnows. On the way we threw the channel catfish to a group of Korean workers on the side of the road. Down the road a little further we saw three Korean children. This was an unusual sight so near the front. We stopped to talk with them.

"Chocolat - have - a - yes?" they asked. We had none. One of them sighted the can of minnows.

"Ah - chop - chop!" We gave them the can of minnows and they divided them among themselves.

"Metcho - have - a - yes?"

"What do they want?" asked a corpsman.

"A match, I guess," I said. We handed the boys a handful of wooden matches. Each of the three children lit a match, held it under a minnow until it stopped wiggling, then chewed the thing whole.

As we drove off, one of the boys called after us, "Numba - one - chop chop!"

Malaria was quite prevalent in Korea. In the early part of the war a large number of returnees were infected with the malarial parasite. Latent malaria was becoming apparent throughout the country. This led to much research on the prevention and treatment of the disease. The results of our program during the summer months of 1952 should have been ample reward for the scientists labor. We rarely saw a case of malaria. As is generally known today, malaria is transmitted to humans by a mosquito. The parasites, in the saliva of the mosquito, are injected into the bloodstream through the mouthparts of the female mosquito as she feeds on the blood.

The medical officer must have a basic knowledge of the mosquito's living habits in order to control this infection. A mosquito can breed only in the presence of water. Rice paddies and other stagnant water must be drained or covered with an oil - DDT film. The drainage of rice paddies in low valleys is no easy task. The length of time it takes an egg to develop into a mosquito is about a week. Thus, in order for a DDT spray to be at all effective, it must be used at least once a week. We were supplied with 5% DDT in a fuel oil mixture. This was transformed into a very effective fog by a tefa machine mounted on a truck, or in the open door of a helicopter. In areas where rice paddies were plentiful, daily spraying was necessary for proper control of mosquitoes. This was especially true

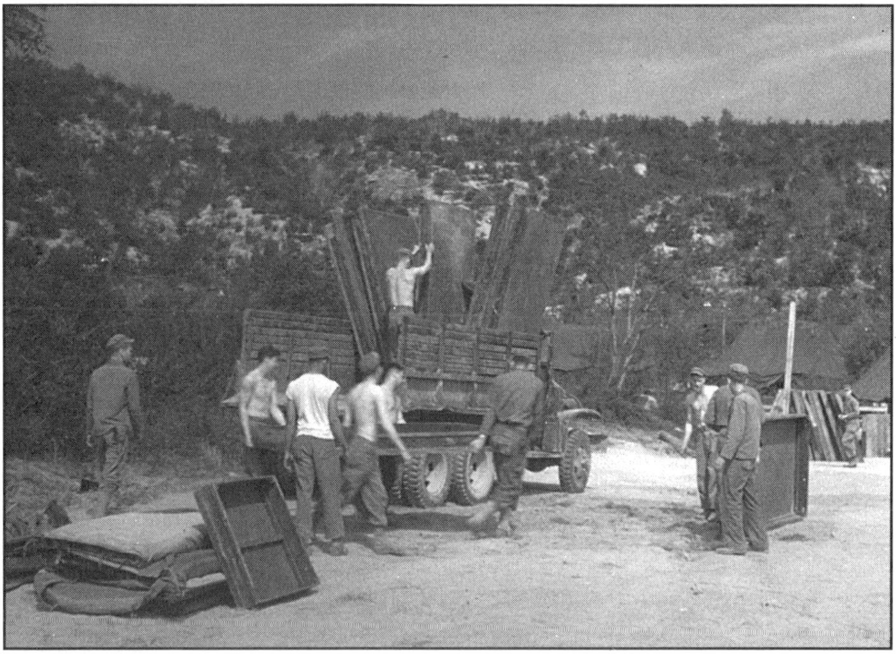

Corpsmen unloading a Janesway hut.

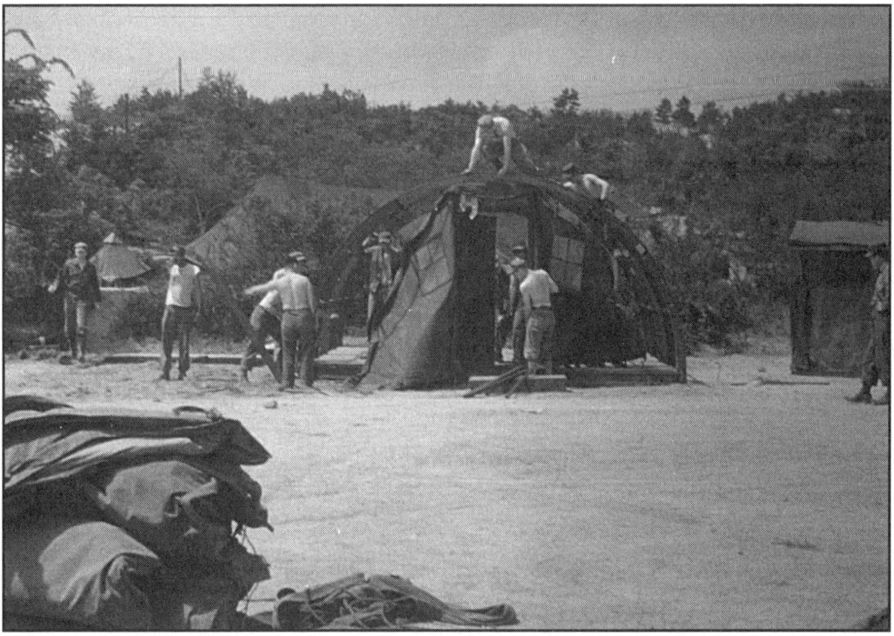

Corpsmen erecting a Janesway hut. The temperature was in excess of 100 degrees.

when the evening breeze increased the flight range of the insect.

On the front line, the marines had to rely on individual protection rather than area control. Protective clothing with long sleeves, and trousers with leggings were worn during the evening hours. These leggings were of a color that looked more yellow than olive drab, or at least they appeared yellow to the enemy, for they referred to the marines as Yellow Legs. Aerosol insecticides proved to be highly effective in tents and bunkers. The mosquito netting was next to food, clothing and armament and was the most valuable item of equipment during the summer months. Without it, proper rest was next to impossible, or at least it was for me. I quite literally detested mosquitoes. The importance of mosquito netting and its proper usage was often difficult to impress upon the enlisted personnel. What a pleasure it was for me to hop into my sleeping bag, tug the mosquito netting underneath the sides, give a couple of blasts with the DDT aerosol bomb to kill any culprits that might have sneaked in while I was doing the tucking, and settle back to listen to the frustrated little varmits sing curses to me from outside.

One of the easiest ways to contract malaria is to associate with Korean natives during the evening hours. A large percentage of them in the area were infected with malaria. I prohibited natives from attending our open air movies. This so-called "front line movie", by the way, is worthy of special note. Movies, of course, were shown only when we were in reserve and thus not really "front line movies". The follies of technical failure coupled with the running commentary by the audience were more entertaining than the movies themselves. All films were shown after dark, and in the open. The projector and screen were set up in a well-protected area, usually behind a hill so that there would be no chance of the enemy seeing the light. The electrical source was from a portable generator which, when placed close at hand, did an outstanding job of drowning out the sound track.

Evenings in Korea were usually cool, even during the hottest of weather, and it was routine to wear a sweater or a field jacket. A few of the more practical enlisted men brought their sleeping bags to the movies. These guys would keep quite comfortable throughout the showing by climbing into their sleeping bags and moving into a semirecumbent position. One hand remained free to handle the cigarettes, candy bars and beer. Up front, in close proximity to the screen, an oil drum was placed for collecting empty beer cans. No one ever thought of quietly placing a beer can at his side until after the show with such a wonderful target up ahead. Thus, throughout the movie, there was a steady clanging of cans and occasionally a burst of cheering when someone accidentally hit the target.

The dogs in Korea loved the movies. I well remember a large black dog, about the size of a shepard, who had spent his entire life with the battalion. He never missed a movie. As a matter of fact, if he was a little late, Blackie's absence would be the topic of conversation. He had a spe-

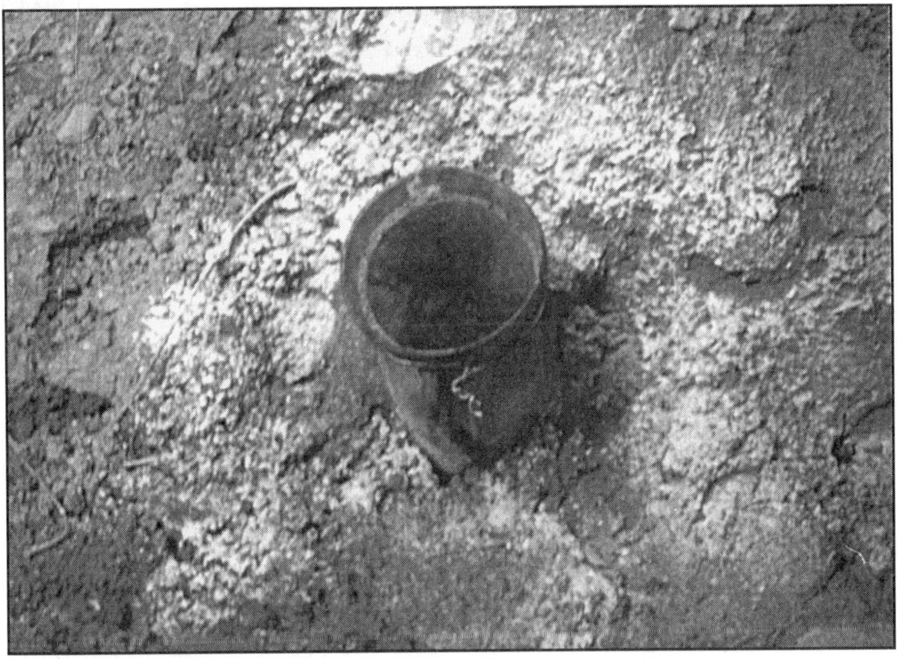

A urinal which is constructed from a used shell. The area is dusted with lime and the top of the shell covered with a screen.

cial spot away from the line of beer can fire and would actually fight if another dog came within reach of a couple of yards. He was otherwise a very gentle animal. I wonder what sort of fascination he associated with motion pictures. During the movie he would remain very quiet as a rule, but occasionally, when the screen action became noisy, he would let go with a long, high pitched howl. As he approached dog adulthood, however, he did this much less frequently, for each howl meant a couple of beer cans thrown in his direction.

Interruptions in the showings were frequent. This was unavoidable for there were just too many sources for trouble. The generator could fail or it could run out of gasoline. The light in the projector frequently burned out. On occasion there were alerts which sent us all scrambling into foxholes and bunkers. When it rained a few would retreat for cover, but not many. During a movie, a film break was a rule rather than the exception. The changing of reels gave us a five minute break. On beer nights, this interruption was well utilized. I had placed several urinal tubes in our movie area, but all for naught, for the guys just couldn't wait their turn. In fact, they completely ignored them in spite of repeated warnings from the commanding officer. They would line up at the edge of the clearing. In unison they produced a sound analogous to a small waterfall.

After the movie, the comments by the enlisted men were as entertaining as the movie itself. Being a doctor, I had the privilege of listening to many conversations which were not curbed by the presence of a line officer. For example, after a movie one evening, I walked away with two enlisted men. I remained quiet while they did the talking.

"Hey, Louis, how'd you like the show?"

"Aww," was the sullen answer.

"Didn't you like the part where Gary Cooper was smoochin' with that dame?"

"Aww."

"What's the matter wit' you? Ya turnin' into a dogface gook or somethin'?"

"Nahh."

"Maybe ya wish you wuz back Stateside under the thumb of Harry Truman. You got rocks?"

"Ah, your mudder wears boondockers. I'll go home when my rotation comes around and not before. What started you flingin' your big yap?"

"Me? Listen to whose talkin'. I'm tryin' to talk about the show, what do I get outta you, but a couple of burps maybe."

"Your friggin' fadder saves beer cans."

"Goodnight, Doc."

At this point I continued on to the shelter with a smile.

The thought of inspecting bunkers always brings to mind one of the many visits by an officer from the rear. The visiting brass from the rear were usually well-received and often gave many helpful suggestions to those doing the fighting - they had been there in the past. Occasionally, an officer would come up for some sort of an inspection, which was obviously uncalled for and not at all appreciated, especially by the front line officers who were required to serve as escorts. I really don't think they had any interest in the activities or had any constructive thoughts. They simply wanted to nose around in order to be able to report on "what I saw on the front line today".

One day a short, rather chubby major came up to the MLR in the morning for the purpose of inspecting bunkers. It was early in the spring, just after the last snow had melted. The major was quite well-dressed for the occasion with helmet, flack jacket, "45 and cane" which we all referred to as an "eatie-wa stick". The inspecting party consisted of a second lieutenant from his staff, plus a lieutenant and two enlisted men from the line. As he walked from bunker to bunker, he found fault with every little detail. He really didn't have a civil word to say to anyone.

The party came to a small two-man bunker on the reverse side of a hill from the MLR. Outside this bunker stood a marine who was brushing off his fatigues and wiping dirt from his face.

"What's your name, son?" the major asked.

"Corporal Cooligan, sir."

"Look at you! You're a disgrace to the Marine Corps! Don't you have any pride in your personal appearance?"

"Yessir!"

"Just because you're on the line is no reason to be as filthy as you are!"

"This is soot, sir. We..."

"Never mind excuses! Consider yourself on report!" (This remark always gave me a laugh. What could be worse than being on the front line?)

It seems that Corporal Cooligan and his buddy, Private First Class Harwood, had been working on their little pot-bellied stove. It had been quite cool that morning and they were lighting it for a little extra heat. During the process of lighting the stove, they accidentally pulled loose the overhead pipes and were instantly covered with soot.

The major poked his head into the bunker,"Your bunker is probably as filthy as you are, Cooligan!"

Then he spied Private Harwood inside.

"Look at you! Come out of there, ya filthy marine!"

Out walked Harwood. His fatigues were covered with soot. The soot, however, did not show on his face and hands, for he was really a black person. The silence was broken when, a few minutes later, some incoming rounds ended the major's inspection. He forgot about putting anyone on report and headed back to the rear. Several months later, a line officer told me that the major had not been in the vicinity of the front line since the incident.

Waste disposal is of utmost importance in the field. Without proper waste disposal, the control of intestinal and insect-born diseases is impossible. Insects and rodents feed on waste. Insects breed on waste. Pathogenic bacteria thrive in waste. Offensive odors are produced by improperly handled waste.

During troop movements, human excreta is disposed of by the digging of a hole. This is covered by several inches of earth. It is time and labor saving to dig a trench during short troop halts. The trench is covered just before troop movement again commences.

On the front, when the line is relatively stable, each company digs a four to six foot deep hole, which is covered with a portable "one-seater" or a homemade job constructed from a wooden crate. During the insect season, this size "head" can be protected by a frame and mosquito netting.

To the rear, from the company, and up to Division Headquarters, larger and more comfortable "heads" are constructed. The site must always be at the opposite end of the camp from the galley and the mess hall. It is situated so as not to drain into the water supply. A four or five foot square, six feet deep hole is dug and covered by a four seater portable fly-tight box. The box is enclosed by a screened wooden framework and covered by a roof.

During the summer, the head sites are changed every two months. We conformed to a bi-daily DDT spraying of our heads. Each morning at about ten o'clock, after the post-breakfast parade, the heads were burned out by the head detail. About a quart of fuel oil was poured into the head. This saturated the paper in a few seconds and a match was dropped into the hole. This procedure prolonged the life of the heads and cut the offensive odor. If the seat covers of any of the heads were left down, this smudge fire would not flare up. I never saw or heard of any of the heads being destroyed by this sanitary measure. Occasionally, one of the guys would absentmindedly sit down, not realizing that the head was being burned out. This resulted in what might be called a "hot seat", but no real harm.

You can be sure that the night visits to these heads were few and far between. Most everyone trained themselves to perform the necessary functions during light hours. Because of odor, drainage, and other sanitary reasons, the heads were placed at some distance from the living area. Now, if you can imagine a frightened figure gropingly making his way through the darkness, with rifle in hand or a hand on his side arm, and toilet paper in the other, you have the picture. The figure reaches the head and looks in all directions before slowly opening the screen door. Once inside, he again looks in all directions through the screen. It was against regulations to put a round in the chamber of a gun in the regimental camp area, unless an order was given to do so or an emergency arose, but I'll bet there were few who made this after dark visit who did not put a round in the chamber of their rifle or pistol. Once the gun is loaded, he slowly lowers his pants and underwear. He again surveys the darkness before sitting down. There is no hesitation or novel reading during this visit. He wouldn't be there in the first place unless it was absolutely necessary. When he finished, the above-mentioned precautionary measures were repeated in reverse order. The first part of the journey back to the living area is one of the slowest and most cautious. As he nears the area, this is abruptly changed to a fast walk or a run, that is, until he is within ten yards or so of the living area. Here he unloads his gun, breathes a sigh and begins a slow gait. He might even be whistling at this point. Someone will ask, as he enters his tent or bunker, "Where ya been, Sam?"

"Oh, just to the head," he answers nonchalantly.

Urine soakage pits are a must in the camp area. They are referred to unofficially as "P-tubes". Without them, offensive odors can readily get out of hand. It may be of interest to the reader to learn how these soakage pits are constructed. First, a hole four feet deep and square is dug and partially filled with broken stone. When the hole is about half-filled with stone, a shell casing, the head of which has been removed, transforming it into a pipe, is set in and held in place by the adding of more stones. When the hole is about filled, the stones are covered with a layer of gravel. A real fancy job is obtained by placing layers of bransack, lime and earth over the gravel. A screen over the end of the shell casing completes the job.

I experimented with these soakage pits attempting to prolong their serviceable life by pouring various mixtures of fuel oil and gasoline into the shell casings. We burned out the heads with good results, why not the pits? But the results were poor and ended in either ignition failure or minor blasts.

Liquid waste and sewage passed from the galley through grease traps and into soakage pits. The grease traps served to prevent cloggage of the soakage pits, and were burned at least once daily, when not in sight of the enemy. The bulldozer made disposal of rubbish and garbage an easy task.

Man's intimate "friend", the rat, and I had our first close association in Korea. The Korean rat, or at least the variety which nightly invaded our camp sites, resembled mostly the brown rat (Rattus Norvegicus). It had a heavy body, short ears, and a tail not as long as many other species. It is written in our field manual, "These animals prefer a diet of grain, vegetable and fruit." Our friends preferred candy bars. They never showed their twitchy noses during the light hours except during the rainy season, when we caught glimpses of them scampering for higher ground.

In general, the rats did no harm other than steal our food and keep us awake at night. As far as we knew, they carried no disease. The smaller field mouse, on the other hand, was labeled as a carrier for hemorrhagic fever.

Our candy bar supply was always much in excess of our appetites. There were no adequate storage places in our tents or bunkers. We tried hiding them in cardboard or wooden boxes. This turned out to be worse than leaving them in the open, for sleep was next to impossible with the constant gnawing and scratching. Either way, they got the candy. Height was no problem for the rat. If he couldn't climb to the candy, a running start and a jump would usually do the trick. The air-tight metal ammunition boxes worked well, but the rats still came around hunting each night. Besides, these metal boxes were hard to come by and made excellent coke and beer coolers when buried. One solution was quite obvious. Why not dispose of all excess candy? We would have done this except for the fact that candy was more valuable than money when dealing with the South Koreans. A few candy bars made the difference between a puttering South Korean and one accomplishing an average day's work.

The rat is an intelligent animal. Why show his face during the day? He would be an easy target, and besides, the days were too hot. Like the enemy ahead of us, he slept during the day in nice cool holes in the ground, and came out only when it was cool and dark. He is quick to learn that where man lives, there is also food. He also knows he is quite safe in the dark, and pays no attention to vocal utterances. A light shown on him only scatters him out of sight or sets him poised to dodge a thrown object. He seemed to know we would not shoot at him in the dark. The shot might attract the attention of the enemy or the missile might ricochet, striking a fellow being. Some of us got fairly skilled at knife throwing.

It was such an occasion to capture a rat by the trapping method, that while in one reserve area, we built a small rat graveyard. The requirement for admission into this cemetery was "death as a result of the rat trap." Each buried rat had a tombstone with a epitaph such as, "One rat, gook type", "Rattus Gookus", "Unknown rat KIA" and the like. At the end of a six-week period, however, there were only about a half-dozen tombstones. I'm sure many of these deaths could be classified as accidental.

The standard Navy oil-cereal rodenticides were quite effective against the rats, that is, when we could get them to eat it. Why they refused to eat these preparations and how they realized it was poisoned is beyond me. Grain is said to be a favorite dish of the rat and the poison was colorless and odorless. In desperation, I went to the mess sergeant and acquired a few cans of peanut butter. With this and the rat poison, we made a water pail full of lethal peanut butter balls. For a while the rats were fooled by these little deathballs and our trouble at night decreased. After a few weeks, however, the number of untouched morsels gradually increased. Then we had another brainstorm. Why not wrap the peanut butter balls to simulate candy bars? This technique was still working beautifully when I departed from the land of mountains and warfare a couple of months later. I must admit, however, the problem of being awakened at night occasionally by a group of rats playing around my sleeping bag was never completely solved.

A doctor on the front must be something of a psychiatrist. Only twenty percent of all psychiatric problems, who were evacuated from Korea and received therapy at a base hospital in Japan, were salvageable for further active duty. The psychiatrists had definitely proved that if these psychiatric casualties were treated at the front, most of them readily adjusted and again became useful fighting men, to say nothing of their adjustment to civilian life in the future. The farther they were evacuated from the front, the more fixed became their mental disturbances. It is for this reason that the military forces placed psychiatrists near the front lines. It might be of interest to cite a couple of examples in order to demonstrate to the reader what can be done with problems on the front.

During a night battle, I received a boy of small stature and of Spanish descent, at the forward aid station. He was unmanageable, raving, and completely unaware of his surroundings. Having no time for a wrestling match, we gave him a potent injection. In a short time, he was fast asleep and the corpsmen carried him back to the sick bay where he remained in his sack for two days, except for visits to the head. Attempting to delve into his past, I contacted his platoon leader. He had been well-adjusted before the battle and was very popular in his platoon as a guitar player.

During the evening of his third day with us, I had a corpsman bring him to my tent. We were drinking beer and singing to the tune of Hagaroo Hank's guitar. In a short time, Hagaroo Hank handed the boy his guitar and asked him to play. This he did without saying a word. It wasn't long before he began singing with us. A few beers put him into a talkative mood and he soon got whatever in particular was bothering him out of his system. The next morning he was anxious to get back to his outfit.

Early one morning, we received a stretcher case, said to be completely paralyzed below the waist line. I went over him carefully and found no injuries. His legs were insensitive to pain, but all his reflexors were normal. We tried every trick in the book to prove him a faker. Two marines from his outfit were at hand and informed us of his paranoid-like personality. Other than his brief and hesitant answers, I found him to be entirely rational.

"You know, Stanley, there is really nothing wrong with your legs. You can walk. Why don't you stand up now and give it a try?"

"Oh no, Doc! The legs are numb. I can't walk!"

I could see we were getting nowhere fast, especially with the presence of the usual curious spectators. The corpsmen carried him to a tent and placed him in a sack, where he proceeded to bathe in his own excretions. During a lull the following evening, I had him carried to the sick bay tent, had him cleaned and bathed, propped up in a chair, and left strict orders that we were not to be disturbed.

As Stanley sat there viewing my every move, I proceeded to file a scratch in the neck of a vial of sodium amytal (truth serum), break off the top of the vial and suction its contents into a hypodermic needle.

"What are you going to do with that, Doc?"

"Nothing at present. Suppose we go over what was happening when

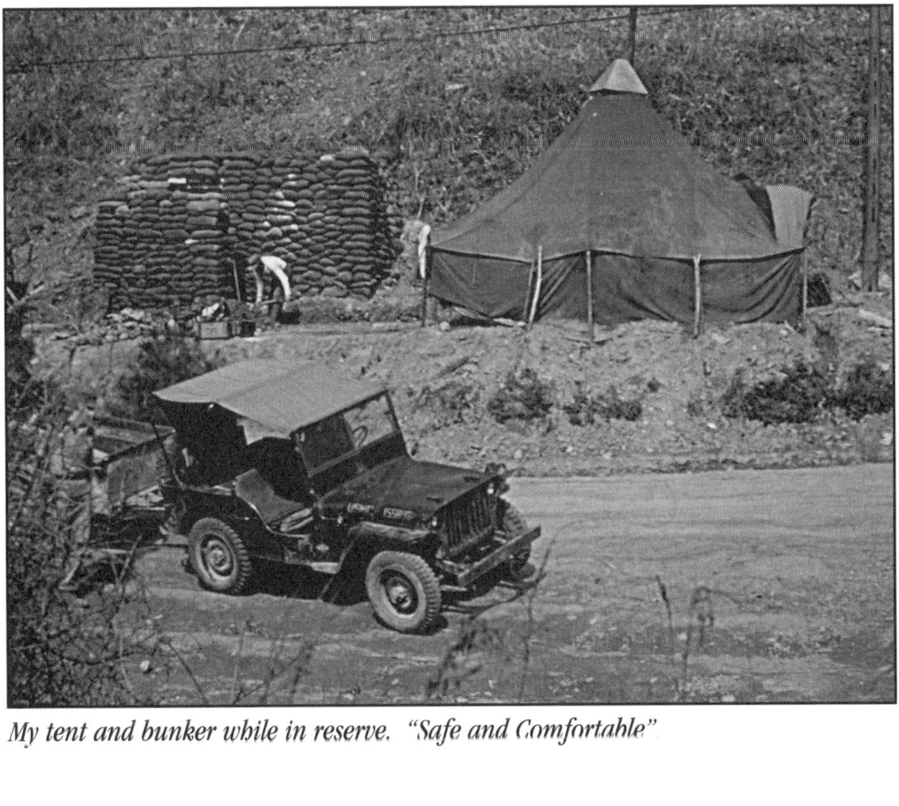

My tent and bunker while in reserve. "Safe and Comfortable"

your legs became paralyzed. You haven't been in Korea long, have you?"

"No, sir, only ten days. I was out on patrol when it happened. They had to carry me back."

"Did you run into any fighting on this patrol?"

"No."

"Look, Stanley, we are pretty sure there is nothing organically wrong with your legs. Something is not clicking right in your brain. Of course, there is always the possibility that you are a faker, but I doubt it. The psychiatrists tell me you will get the best result if you are treated right here. Now, I have something in the syringe to relax you. It will help us to get at whatever is bothering you. I'm going to leave the decision to you. I want you to give this a try, otherwise, I prefer not to waste my time with further words. What do you say?"

"I'm not a coward, Doc. I'll take the stuff. You'll see I'm not faking!"

I then began the intravenous injection of sodium amytal. Stanley relaxed immediately and began to talk.

"All the guys think I'm a coward, don't they, Doc? They think I'm putting on just so I won't have to be out front. Well, I'm not."

"Just relax now, Stanley."

A little more of the amytal slurred his speech. The dosage was now adequate, so I removed the needle

"Where are you from, Stanley?"

"New Jersey."

"Did you go through high school?" I asked.

"Yes."

"Play any sports?"

"No."

"How did you get along with the other fellows in high school?"

"Not too well."

"Why, Stanley?"

"Because of my religion."

"What had your religion go to do with it?"

"You know, alot of guys don't associate with the Jewish."

"What have you done since high school?"

"Nothing. They drafted me."

"Ever been away from home before?"

He began to weep, so I let him go at it and smoked a cigarette. When he had calmed down a little I asked, "How do you get along with the fellows in your outfit?"

"The same way. They are all Protestants and Catholics. They don't like the Jewish. I stay by myself most of the time."

I thought. This may be the answer. He has a feeling of inferiority and is in a situation where he believes himself unwanted. It must be quite a knock trying to cope with a situation where there is a definite possibility of being killed or wounded and at the same time feeling unwanted.

"I can truly sympathize with you, Stanley. On the other hand, you have to meet people half way to acquire friendships. A share of the difficulty lies with the other fellows, I am sure, but you should make certain advances. Do you have a buddy in the outfit?"

"No."

"I'll speak to your platoon leader and have him look out for you and fix you up with a buddy. You're supposed to have one, you know."

"No, I can never go back with that platoon," he insisted.

"All right. Here's what I'll do. I have a personal friend who is a company commander in another battalion. I'll get you transferred to his company with his promise to look out for you. Now, will you try to walk for me?"

"Sure, I'll try to walk. I've tried before. I want to walk, but I just can't."

I helped him to his feet and let him go. He swayed back and forth but did not fall. During the next half hour I tried my level best to make him take a step. All attempts were in vain. He just would not walk. I smoked another cigarette and went at him again.

Stanley was still unable to take a step two hours after the injection of sodium amytal. By this time, he was quite alert from my continuous questioning and pleading. I was ready for the sack. He could stand and sit without aid. Feeling the need for a breath of fresh air and maybe a little nip, I took a walk to my tent and came back with a fifth of whiskey. I offered Stanley a drink.

"Sure, Doc, I'll take a drink as long as you're having one, too."

One drink led to another. At about one o'clock in the morning we walked out of the sick bay, arm in arm. Stanley had found a friend. He staggered in the direction of the urinal, and I in the direction of my tent. I do believe he could walk better than I.

I met Stanley a few weeks later, standing guard for his new outfit. He again thanked me for a pleasant evening.

When the enemy was not beating on us, we ran out of activities to occupy our time and things to talk about. To compensate for this, we invented various types of amusement, such as pitching washers into a tin can (we had no pennies). Joe Sharpe taught me how to blow spit bubbles. Try it sometime. It takes endless hours of practice. We devised various methods for capturing flies. When it was not too hot and we were ambitious, there was always the contest to see who could dig the deepest foxhole. In my case, I turned to chewing tobacco and raising a "tea strainer". There were many variations of the mustache, beards, goatees, sideburns and the like, but I stuck to the "Barbershop Quartet" style with great success.

Now, the raising of a large mustache has its own problems, especially after the growth has exceeded the lip margins by about an inch. Each morning it must be combed and twisted upwards. Mustache wax was not to be had, so most of us used a low melting point dental wax, which we obtained from "Hagaroo Hank", our regimental dentist.

One day I was on a supply run with two other officers. They were sitting on edge of a stretcher on one side of the jeep ambulance while I occupied a very comfortable recumbent position in a wire mesh stretcher on the opposite side. Seeing the other two smoking, I pulled out my package of cigarettes (unfiltered Camels). Instead of trying to light a match, I borrowed an already burning cigarette from one of the officers. The ambulance hit a bump and the jolt cause me to make contact between the lighted end of the cigarette and my mustache. The resulting flames were so lively that within seconds I was choking on the smoke. Every muscle of my body was instantly alerted. Quick reflexes at a time like this were essential. It was a question of quenching an early fire or suffering the consequences - a burned upper lip.

The driver, by now, had turned to see what was causing such a commotion. A fit of laughter from all three was accompanied by a lurch of the ambulance, and we were all thrown to the floor. While stabilizing the ambulance and again resuming our course on the road, the driver narrowly missed a couple of pedestrians. All this excitement resulted in no damage other than to my now smoldering mustache.

From that day on I was known as "The Mustache That Walks Like a Man."

Chapter Sixteen

YOKE

From time to time I had this strong suspicion that Korea wasn't a peninsula, but rather a floating island which traveled to the Arctic in the winter and the equator in the summer. This hot summer day, June 27, added more validity to my theory than I ever wished. I turned and looked toward the sky, my sunglasses barely making the bright sky visible, as the 10 o'clock flyby of our peace-keeping delegates flew over the camp in their helicopters, headed for Panmunjon.

The temperature, from my best guess, had already reached a hundred, and it wasn't even noon yet. I was sitting, actually squatting, outside the colonel's tent with a few others that had been called for a meeting of special staff. The anticipation was palpable, the sweat was pouring from us in streams, and I had long since given up trying to keep it from running down my face. My only thought was, "I just hope the colonel is making each of us one of his famous martinis, straight up, no ice, one olive." I didn't even have enough water left in me to salivate, but my mouth went through the motions anyway.

Everyone was accounted for and we entered the colonel's tent. The first thing he said and the only thing he had to say was, "We are going to take Yoke tonight." Yoke, that was the code name for a hill more than two miles north of the front line. The colonel studied our faces, gauging our reactions and then continued, "Then if luck is with us, we will swing east and advance our entire line for nearly two miles. There is a good possibility that we will meet some tough opposition, so this little hike is not going to be a bed of roses." The sweat was pouring off the colonels forehead, partly from the heat and the rest from his concerns. He took a deep breath and continued.

"The division commander has ordered me to take this hill. We need the high ground as an outpost for enemy observation." His voice rose as he began to talk in depth on battle maneuvers and fighting tactics with the line officers. It took him more than an hour and a half to complete the briefing. He then said it was the medical officers turn, Tom, Roy, and me.

"I want two of you to cover the rear of the battalion from where we are going to advance. As you have heard, the push will be a U-shaped drive. First, we will climb up and take Yoke, leave a company there, and advance eastward, and then back to our present line."

Tom volunteered to take the east end of the U-drive, which left Roy and I to cover the push-off point.

The meeting disbanded, and Roy, Tom and I headed back to the sick bay area and opened a round of beer from the sunken ammo-box cooler. We all agreed that this was not a night for resting, none of us were going to sleep tonight.

We sat sipping our beers in silence, thinking of what was to come, when Roy finally broke the silence with a thought we all had been thinking.

"I say stay where we are. Why take that ground? It will only end in a bloody mess, on both sides. It will just end up like another '104'."

"104" was a hill we had assaulted a few weeks previously, its memory was still like a fresh wound in our minds, this maneuver resulting in 160 killed or wounded. That twenty-four hour period had been one day that will forever be burned into my brain.

I had become adjusted, as much as I could, to the routine daily number of wounded and usually there was time for meals, sleep, maybe a bull session and a few well earned beers, but with these large operations there was only time for the treatment of the wounded. During a push from morning to night all we did was treat the injured, maybe gulp down a few K-rations in between treatments, and sleep was a luxury we went without. The other doctors and I were not required to move out with troops, but a third of our corpsmen, about eight of ten men, were so instructed. Some volunteered, others had to be ordered and that was one of the many jobs I hated carrying out. During many of these operations the percentage of corpsmen killed or wounded was often greater than that of the fighting Marines.

Our jeep and field ambulances had been gassed, greased, and oiled. I called "wonderful-forward", the field phone call for the helicopters, and asked for three "whirlybirds" to be in readiness for the night. We moved out when the orders came through, my mind intent on what had to be done. One of our chief hospital corpsmen took a jeep and trailer to the rear for additional supplies. It would have been an inexcusable error to run out of supplies since there was always plenty to be had if you only did the asking. Roy and I followed the battalion to the front line, where we were to remain and set up a makeshift first aid station. Tom would be waiting with his crew in a bunker at a point where the Marines would again approach our line, and some of the corpsmen remained at the battalion aid station. The regimental aid station and the medical companies, MASH units, were alerted. We were now as prepared as we could be for whatever might come our way.

We arrived at nine in the evening at a large apple orchard, which was about two hundred yards behind the front line, where we set up the forward aid station. The orchard was in the area called the "corridor" which is the gateway to Panmunjon. The temperature had dropped to a cooler 75 degrees and thankfully there was a full moon in a cloudless sky, so no lights were necessary. Just to the right of the orchard, as we faced enemy ground, was a battalion of Marines. I imagined our presence next to them didn't do much for their morale, but they did know we were close by if they needed us.

I had a wonderful bunch of corpsmen working with me, so it was unnecessary to issue very many orders. As soon as we arrived they went to work, digging foxholes, checking supplies, assembling the wooden horses we needed to support the stretchers. They put the ambulances out of sight under the fruit trees. Roy and I checked our wire communications. We had three lines: one was to Tom who was not yet situated at his outpost, a second was with battalion headquarters, and the other ran to regimental headquarters where three helicopters were on call to evacuate the more seriously wounded.

After everything was pretty much in place Roy and I stopped to converse, staying near our foxholes, and discussed the situation. For the most part we estimated that the number of casualties we would treat would be well over a hundred. After a while we joined the marine officers.

The marines were much more nervous than we were, and rightfully so, as they waited for zero hour speaking among themselves in hushed tones. I tried in vain, a few times, to lighten the oppressive mood as much as I could with a couple of corny jokes, but all I got was a few chuckles and silence. Nervous as a cat and not ready to stay in one place for too long, I decided to walk among the troops. Studying the fighting marines in a situation such as this absorbed me completely, appealing to my natural investigative side. The various human reactions to an inevitable oncoming battle were as diverse as the differences in the men themselves and held for me a strange fascination.

The typical marine is judged as being a stiff, emotionless, well-trained fighter who follows the manual to the letter and reveres the Marine Corps as a father figure. During these waiting periods, however, the marine is left to the mercy of his own thoughts much the same as a condemned man waiting in his cell for the hopeful mercy of a pardon, in the face of an execution. During this short period of time, as their thoughts tangled with their emotions, many of these marines, most of whom are still boys, were not the well-trained fighting machines they always hoped they'd be. They were humans facing death.

The extremes of emotions were as far different as the sun is to the moon. A few of them seemed fearless, laughing, playing, joking as if they were oblivious to the impending battle and as carefree as children. Others sat alone or paced back and forth. Others were motionless, staring at pictures, hoping they would survive another battle, afraid to face the unknown, and hoping that tonight their number wasn't up.

All too soon ten o'clock came and zero hour was upon us. We wished the officers luck, many of them were friends we had come to know during our many months of close association. I saw Tom Greene, a good friend. He came over and wished me good luck. I offered him a bit of the Beechnut chewing tobacco I had. He took it graciously with a smile and waved as he walked away. I then returned to the area where our foxholes were and waited.

The minutes seemed to drag on for hours. The silence was frightening. It was as if everything was lifeless, nothing moved, except for the mosquitoes, but in the shadows far enough away where we couldn't hear, our troops were approaching their objective, Yoke. I could see in my mind's eye the Marines proceeding single file to the foot of the hill, their figures slightly hidden in the shadows, but visible in the bright moonlight. Then at 10:45 the sounds of battle began.

At first the eerie sounds from the burp guns echoed through the air, followed by the bursting of grenades. In answer to the first bombardment of gunfire we heard carbines, M-1 machine guns, and the echoing sound of more grenades. It was as if a morbid symphony was reaching an increasing crescendo, rising in pitch and intensity until the deafening roar of the mortar and artillery shells joined the deadly cacophony.

"It will be at least a half an hour before we see any casualties," Roy commented, his voice surprisingly loud over the din of battle.

"Guess I'll blow up my "bubble" and recline next to my boudoir for a short nap," I answered, trying to lighten things up a bit.

"You'll be eaten by mosquitoes if you do," Roy answered, chuckling.

I searched deep into a pocket, pulled out my bug repellent, waved it in the air and smiling, rubbed it on all the exposed portions of my skin. Roy followed suit when I had finished and he passed it on to a corpsman. Somehow no one had remembered their mosquito repellent solution, but were more than glad to use mine because the little devils were getting thicker by the minute.

Free from the onslaught of the bugs, I reclined on my air mattress with the thought of relaxing and reducing my nervous tension before the casualties came pouring in. I was lying no more than a foot away from the edge of my foxhole. Well, it wasn't all mine because my sidekicks, HM1 Rector and HM2 Beauchamp did most of the digging. I had been resting on the mattress for less than a minute when Morpheus hit me with a mighty blow and I was fast asleep.

Time passed quickly. In that short time our rocket company,"The Haul-Ass Boys" had quietly advanced and set up within 50 yards of where I was sleeping. Their nickname was perfect, for a company such as this advances into a position, sets up their sights, aims, fires and then disappears as rapidly as they had come.

They fired, and I believe in that instant I lost a few years off of my life. The next thing I knew I was on the bottom of the foxhole, upside down with my helmet pushed into my face, and about half a pound of dirt under my fatigue jacket. I was sure the enemy found out our position and were lobbing shells in our direction. After a while, I finally got rearranged, my heartbeats slowed down to a pace I could at least count, and I popped my head out of the foxhole, yelling at the top of my lungs.

"What the hell's going on?"

I heard laughter and turned to find Roy and the corpsmen doubled over. They had been anticipating my reaction to the rocket fire and had watched me jump out of a deep sleep and fling myself into the foxhole. Obviously they were amused. I soon joined in their laughter and I must say this served to reduce my tension and elevate our spirits.

We waited in silence, but soon from a distance, we heard the noise we were dreading, the rumbling of an armored vehicle, which most assuredly would be carrying the wounded. As the vehicle came closer, we could see that every available space on the surface was occupied by a casualty. A few were sitting, but most were lying still, hanging on the best they could, or being supported by another marine.

We sprung into action. One of the first casualties I came to was such a good friend, when I saw what had happened to him, I did something I had never done before during triage, I experienced emotion. It was Lieutenant Greene, both his legs were missing at the level of the groin, he had been fighting at the head of his company until a mortar exploded nearly beneath him. There was nothing I could do, I felt helpless, I was angry. For the first time I didn't know what I was going to do.

"They are both gone aren't they, Doc?" Tom's voice startled me. I had no idea he had been conscious. I nodded, afraid to open my mouth fearing my voice would crack, heavy with emotion. Tom continued, "Tell my wife and son how it happened."

He then slipped into unconsciousness and died shortly thereafter. As he lay before me, I felt sorry for him, that his life had to end this way, but I felt more sorrow for the ones he left behind, his family back home, who in three days would receive a telegram that would change and overshadow their lives for years.

"The United States Marine Corps regrets to inform you that Lieutenant Thomas Greene was killed in action in western Korea. He had conducted himself in a heroic and courageous manner."

Such small words for a life that had been good and caring. I stood up, ordered a marine to take Tom's body away and managed to suppress everything I was feeling. I would have to wait for another time and another place to mourn, right now I had to save lives, not grieve over the ones that were already lost.

There was an endless river of casualties. Two among them were the corpsmen we had sent out with the troop. As I worked, going from one wounded man to another, a couple of marines came up to me with a stretcher. They were carrying an entire lower body, boots and all. When they asked what they should do with it, all I could do was swear, "God damn it! Put it out of sight and get the hell away from here."

I was furious. Why on earth had they bothered to carry this all the way back to us? Surely this offered no means of identification. Maybe it was a means of getting away from the battle for a while or simply it could have been a buddy of theirs.

Hour after hour, after hour, after hour passed. I was covered in blood. I smelled of it and I was certain I would never be free of it. We had had every conceivable type of wound and more than the usual number of amputations. The shells landing nearby, the overhead airbursts and the thought of a possible enemy overrun were now of little concern to any of us, for every one of our mental and physical efforts were being utilized in the treatment of the wounded.

Three of the whirlybirds were doing their usual efficient evacuation of the seriously wounded to the medical companies. In order to maintain our supply of stretchers, we adhered to the following routine with these helicopters. At the MASH level, corpsmen would remove the two casualties on stretchers from the outborn little capsules on the helicopter. Other corpsmen replaced these with empty stretchers, which were removed when the helicopter returned to us at the front line. The casualties on stretchers were then carried from our saw horses to the helicopters as we finished treatment. I had pictured a ride in the outborn litter capsules to be a frightening ordeal, anything but conducive to the best handling of the wounded soldier, especially when in shock. But, the men had to be moved to get treatment and this was the fastest way.

At two in the morning I noticed one of the newer corpsmen, Sammy, getting that all too familiar look in his eyes. They were glassed over, he seemed haunted, he wouldn't respond when spoken to, and he was unable to move. He had become catatonic and absolutely useless. I led him to a foxhole and told him to remain down there until we were ready to return to the rear. He was in the same position when I went to check on him in the morning.

In the light of day the carnage around us seemed that much more frightening. We were more than a bit weary. Tom had joined us by this time, telling us that the troops never reached his area. We had informed him of our heavy load by field phone, and since our troops were pretty well beaten back, he had left his outpost to lend us a much needed hand.

In the end, the battle of Yoke had been lost. I counted our copy of the evacuation tags, there were 96 wounded, 14 dead and 4 missing. The folks back home would get the usual front page story, "Marines take Yoke" and

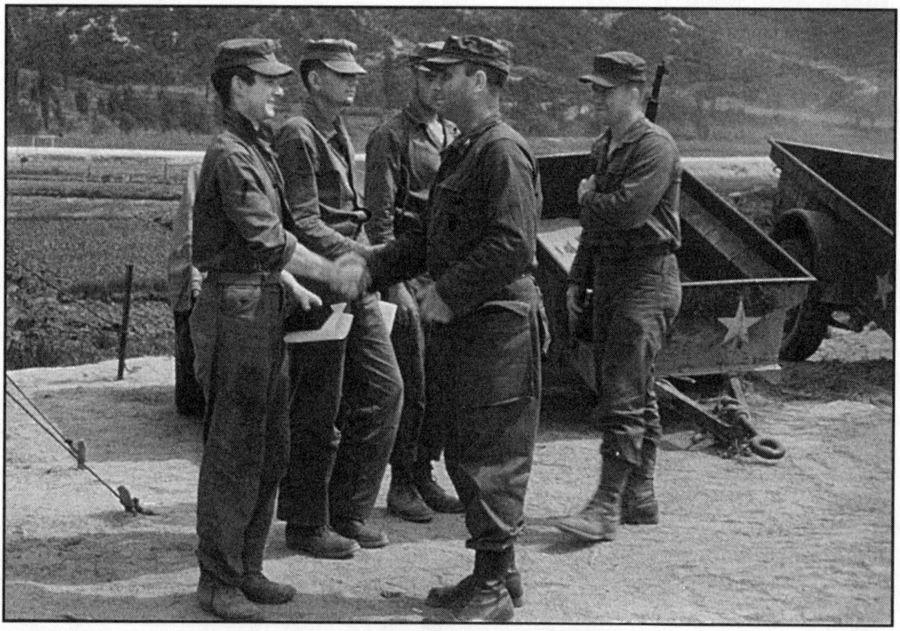

Colonel Honzowitz is awarding putple hearts to three of our men with "minor" shrapnel wounds.

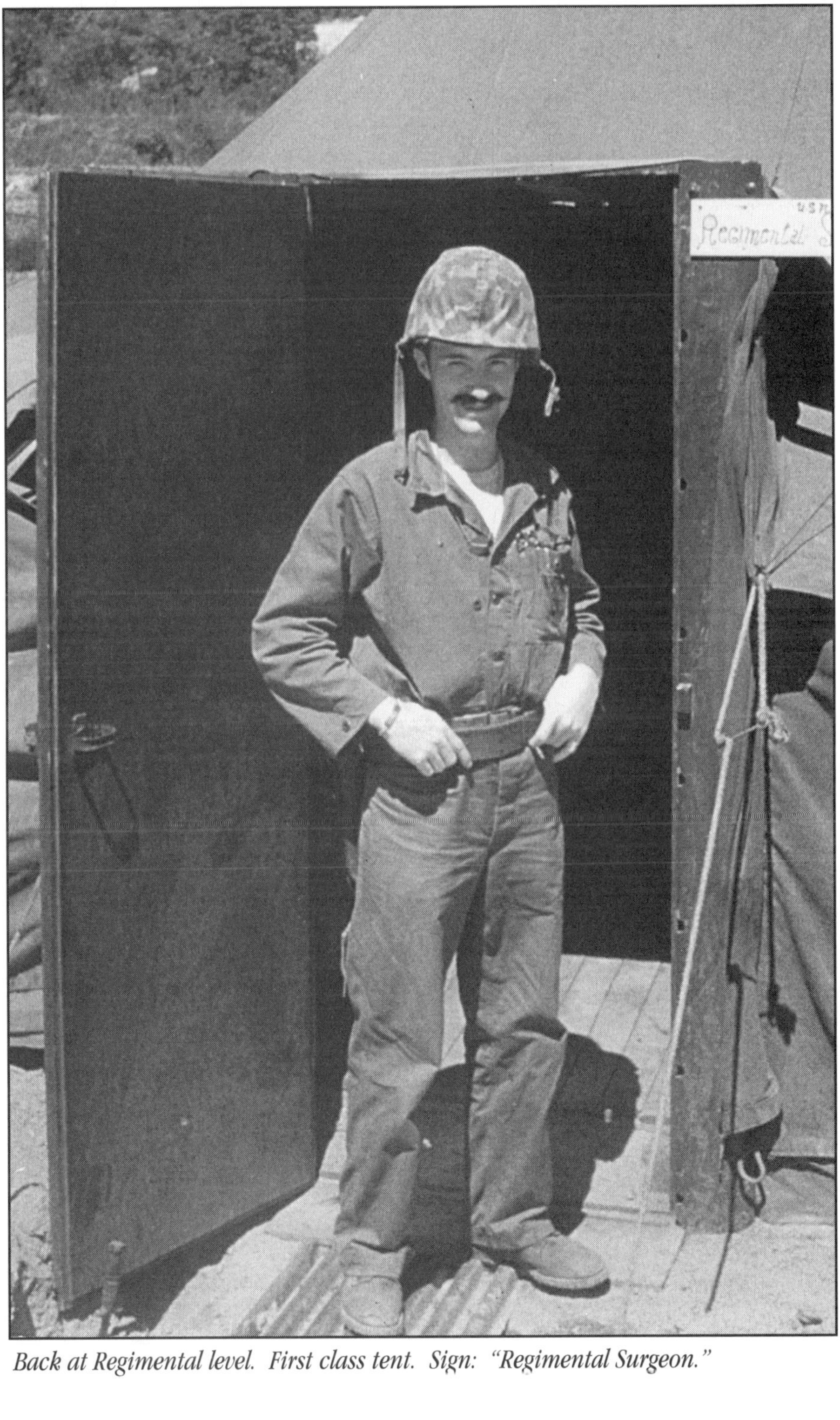

Back at Regimental level. First class tent. Sign: "Regimental Surgeon."

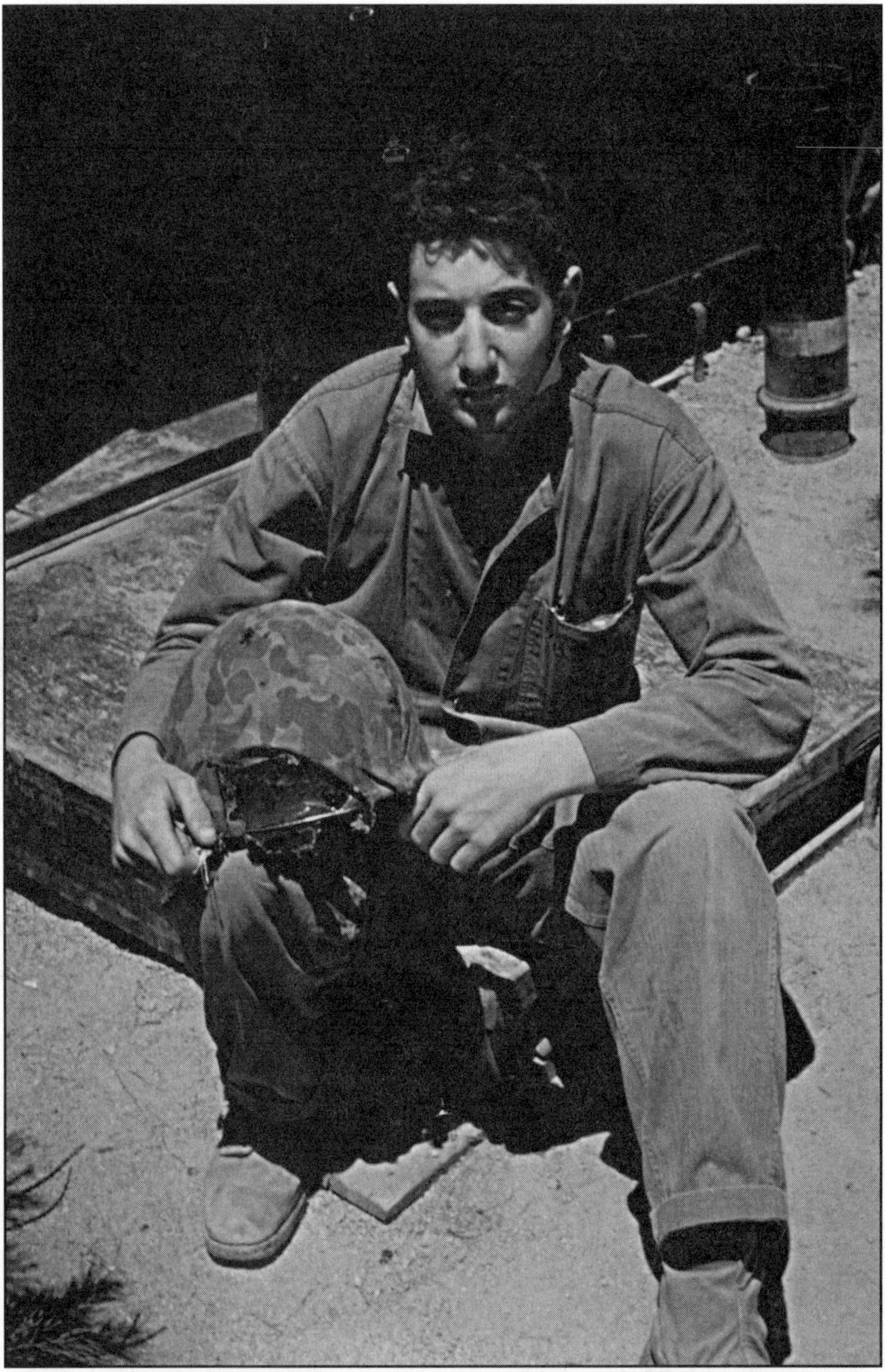

Lucky Marine–A burp gun bullet went through his helmet and spun around inside. The end result was a small wound in his left neck. "You should have heard the racket inside my helmet, Doc."

then in next edition, on about page 7, there would be a small paragraph stating that the marines were pushed from Yoke by an overwhelming number of Chinese troops in a Western Korean scrimmage. Or, perhaps the papers back home wouldn't even mention our activities. A large number of hometown newspapers I had received by mail made no mention of the Korean War.

I rode back to the rear area. Upon entering my tent, I looked into the small mirror we used for shaving, and saw the image of someone I had not previously seen, the face caked in dried blood. I looked at my hands. It was as though I had dipped then in a bucket of blood. My clothes were soaked through with blood, my hat, fatigue tops, pants, shoes, everything - even my underwear. It's a good thing we didn't have AIDS in those days.

I had mixed emotions. We had lost a fight, but I had an inward proud feeling of a job well done. At any rate, we were one day closer to going home. I needed a bath and some sleep.

Bullshit! That is how I felt in 1952. Today, as this is written, it is the 41st anniversary of the end of the Korean War and I don't have mixed emotions. It was a waste of beautiful young lives. Who ordered this ridiculous poke at the enemy? Was it a politician sitting on his fat duff in Washington? War is senseless. There has to be a better way of settling differences.

Chapter Seventeen

CAMP OTSU

It was late summer when I arrived at the First Provisional Casual Company, Fleet Marine Forces in Camp Otsu, Japan. Otsu is a relatively small town situated on the shore of beautiful Lake Biwa with Little Fuji Mountain in the distance, and very close to Kyoto, a large city which until modern times, had been the capital of Japan. It was now the art, religious and cultural center of Japan. Camp Otsu had been one of the training sites for the Japanese Kamikaze, or suicide, pilots. They received a period of intensive training here and then were allowed six weeks of wine, women, and song, or just about anything else they wanted, before going on to an almost certain death. Camp Otsu was an excellent duty spot, as I soon learned.

Our quarters were well-kept and comfortable. The food was excellent. Each morning we had a choice of ham and eggs or steak and eggs. So, you can imagine what the rest of the meals were like.

The marine casualties sent to Otsu were basically those with minor wounds, or others that were recovering rapidly from more serious wounds. At this point, they were not sufficiently disabled to warrant their return to the United States, nor were they well enough so that they could return to active duty in Korea.

Approximately three hundred marine casualties from the Korean War now occupied Camp Otsu. A full bird marine colonel was in charge of the camp. He lived with servants in a beautiful house on a hill toward the back of the camp. Flower gardens surrounded the colonel's quarters and its only access was a long, stone stairway beginning at the camp level. The colonel had a full component of marine officers to run his camp. There was an officer in charge of each camp function: motor pool, mess, communications, officer's club, and the like. He spent most of his time in his house on the hill. I wondered what he did to occupy his time and suspected that he was somewhat depressed being assigned to a position such as this for it meant that he would remain at his present rank until he retired. From time to time he showed up at the officer's club and never seemed to be very sober.

Two rather large barrack-like buildings housed the medical department of Camp Otsu. The crew at the sick bay area consisted of a navy surgical team with three doctors and six corpsmen. They were in navy uniform. There were also seven corpsmen in marine uniform who were Korean casualties. I was also in a marine uniform.

Most of the navy corpsmen were situated in the record department at one end of the sick bay. Here they maintained the health records of all personnel aboard plus those of all transient and missing members of the First Marine Division. Two corpsmen manned the sick call treatment room, one the pharmacy, three the sick bay ward, which was a separate building, and one served as venereal disease control man. The three doctors in navy uniform held sick call each morning and tended to the patients in the sick bay ward. After I had been there a very short time, we all got along very well together and quite efficiently managed the

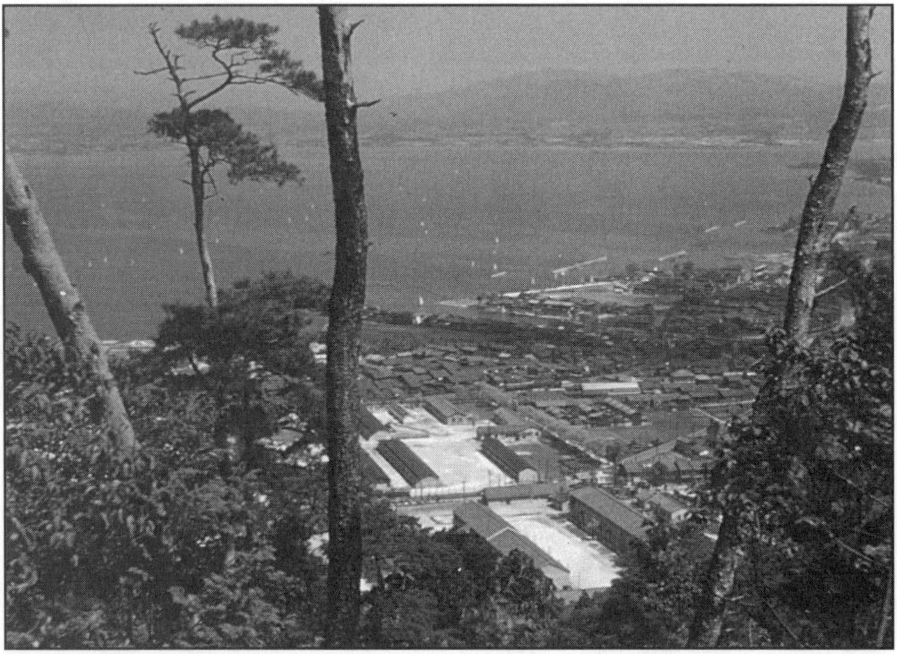

The main medical building at Camp Otsu.

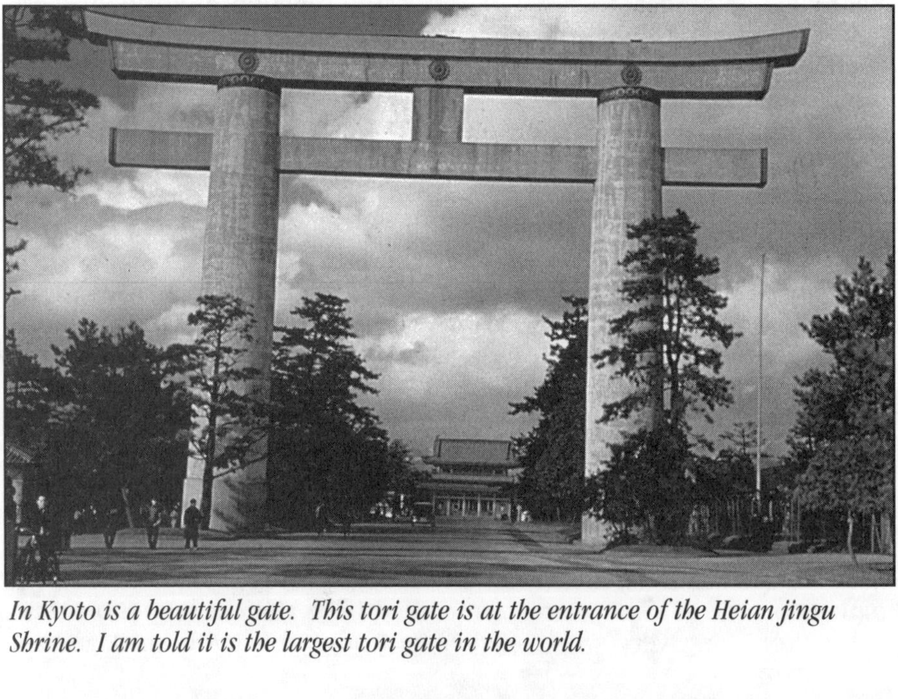

In Kyoto is a beautiful gate. This tori gate is at the entrance of the Heian jingu Shrine. I am told it is the largest tori gate in the world.

department as a group.

As marine medical officer in charge it was my duty to classify the marine casualties, regardless of rate or rank, as they were discharged from the hospital in Tokyo, and during their stay at Camp Otsu. There were three groups in this classification. "A" group was ready for duty in Korea. Members of this group were returned to their outfits in Korea after a short period of reconditioning. "B7-B30" (numerals designating the number of days) became temporary members of the casualty company and were assigned to various departments. At the end of the "B" period, each was reclassified. If the marine had not completely recuperated from his wounds, another "B" duty was in order. "B45" would literally translate as "unfit for duty within 45 days". Actually this was a one way ticket to the United States. Most marines coming aboard knew the meaning of a "B45". Some would ask, "What are my chances for a B45, Doc?" but not many. I suspect that these were not real marines, but rather those that had been drafted and then transferred to the Marine Corps.

The corpsmen were always a source of entertainment for me. Almost all of them had a purple heart ribbon on their blouse, if they wore ribbons. HM2 Capshaw was my right-hand man and a perpetual wit. One side of his face looked like someone had tinted it with charcoal, the result of a mortar blast. The fine shrapnel and dirt had tattooed the left side of his face. Each marine coming into my office was introduced by Capshaw as, "Doctor, approaching one head, jar type". As I mentioned, marines are often referred to as jarheads because of their haircuts.

Capshaw seldom went by his given name during his stay in Camp Otsu for he had been given a nickname by the Japanese. Capshaw's eyebrows were thick, black and met in the midline. Thus, the Japanese called him "Ichi Mangi-San," which in English means one eyebrow. Ichi Mangi-San saw to it that I was never in want. For example, we were having difficulty obtaining heat for the sick bay from our source, an army heating plant 300 yards away from our campsite. He provided me with a hibachi - a Japanese pottery piece in which charcoal is burned, and a large bag of charcoal. The marines must have thought we were rather soft-headed as we sat on the floor around the hibachi discussing their cases. The hibachi, by the way, indirectly obtained action, and thus heat from the army major in charge of the army heating plant. Our colonel raised hell with him when he learned of the primitive heat source in my office.

HM2 Stanley went by the nickname of "Rip Van Winkle". Rip had been out on the town one evening and consumed much beyond his capacity of beer. The following morning he assumed the duty of Mate of the Day. One function of the Mate of the Day is to keep the daily log. He opened the log correctly with "On March 4..." His hangover must have become progressively more severe as the day passed for when he turned the page, he dated it "December 7." To make an almost unbelievable story, he signed out at the end of the day with "September 7." Rip never noticed his mistakes until they were pointed out to him the next day by an angry Chief.

HM3 Smith manned the pharmacy. Here he filled prescriptions coming from sick call, examined blood, and venereal disease smears. He also kept the pharmacy log. On the far end of one shelf, away from the mess of the pharmacy, Smith kept a number of unlabeled bottles. These contained flavorings he had brewed from oranges, lemons, raisins, apricots, spices and the like. Their usage in his tea concoctions led to his nickname, "The Tea Man". Each afternoon at about 2 o'clock, I could expect a mug of tea, the likes of which I had never before tasted. He appeared as a mad chemist adding bits of various flavorings with a medicine dropper as he stood over the steaming beaker of tea.

The Tea Man was also known for his practical jokes. A marine sergeant named Ragan appeared at the sickbay complaining of abdominal cramps. The pain was not localized, not acute and he was without other symptoms. To rule out parasitic infection, I asked him to bring in a stool sample for microscopic examination. Ragan started to balk at the request, but looked at me and said, "yessir". I was wearing a marine uniform with officer's insignia - he had no choice. Ragan returned the same afternoon with a specimen for the Tea Man.

Smitty prepared a slide and said, "Hey Doc! Come on over here and look at this!"

Sure enough, Ragan had ascaris lumbricoides. I asked Ragan to report for worm treatment. I didn't see him coming the next morning for I was occupied with another patient. The Tea Man called to him as he passed the pharmacy.

"Hey, Ragan, got worms, eh?"

"So I heard. Did you see them?"

"Sure, come on in. I'll show you one."

The Tea Man handed Ragan a bottle. Ragan took a look at it and slumped to a chair in a semi-faint. HM3 Smith had found a 3 inch green centipede running around outside the dispensary.

HM3 Baird was, among other names, "The Poet". His productions might have been much more worthy had he concentrated a bit on what he was doing rather than his affinity for speed and volume. At least, three times a week, The Poet entered my office, bowed, uttered a Japanese greeting, handed me one of his works of art and departed. I salvaged a few of these and placed them in my diary after they had been disseminated through the enlisted barracks. For instance:

MOVING ON, CAMP OTSU STYLE

<u>Morning Verse</u>

A big Marine going down the walk,
He ain't very sick but he sure will squawk.
He's feeling bad.
He's "A" duty and trying a shrewdie.
He's feeling bad.
"I've told you, doctor, from time to time,

That I can't march with this twisted spine.
I'm feeling bad.
I've got a headache and that ain't no fake.
I'm feeling bad.
I've got a bad cold with a terrible cough,
My poor old arms are about to drop off.
I'm feeling bad.
My feet are flat, I can't go back. (to Korea)
I'm feeling bad.
<u>Evening Verse</u>
Seventeen hundred (5 p.m.) and he's feeling fine.
He has an Otsu Queen on his mind.
He's liberty bound.
He has two thousand yen on liquour to spend.
He's liberty bound
One beer down and he takes a stand.
For this Korean War he is just the man.
He's mighty brave.
He'll get him a "star" with his B.A.R. (rifle)
He's mighty brave.

Torii Toyojira was the Japanese janitor for the sick bay. We all called him "Papa-San". You will note the suffix, "San" after Japanese names and nicknames. It is absolutely essential. The omission of San is a rude and ignorant error. Papa-San was proud of his American nickname. Usually it is the function of the corpsmen to swab the decks, scrub and polish the furniture. This was not the case at Camp Otsu Sick Bay. We all contributed a few cents a week to Papa San's salary, enough to keep him and his large family quite comfortable.

Papa-San was a tiny man with dainty features. He was, without doubt, what an American would consider a handsome Japanese. I guess his age to be about sixty-five. He was probably much older.

Each morning Papa-San would be waiting for me in my office, with mop in hand. "U-sssss," he would say along with a low bow. I answered him in Japanese, for he spoke no English other than "yes" and "thank you". Never a day passed that he did not wet-mop our unvarnished floors. We all tried to impress upon him that an interval of three days would be quite adequate, for the daily mopping made the sick bay damp. The soft wood floors were rotting with such treatment. Besides, Papa-San was too old for such labor. Speak as we would, scold and plead, Papa-San continued his mopping. Later on I learned through an interpreter that Papa-San thought his few dollars-a-month salary very high and felt honor-bound to mop the floor each morning.

The patients frequently provided us with a bit of humor. One example is the saga of a tall, thin, blond lad with an expressionless face, a hillbilly gait, and a southern accent. He was straight from the hills of South

Carolina. He reported aboard early one morning for classification and I examined his health record. He had had moderate frostbite of both feet and was by directive, automatically unfit for further Korean duty. Having completed the rounds from Korea, hospital ship and Navy hospital, he was now ready for classification and transportation to the States. I saw a vision defect noted in his health record. It said, "wears glasses."

"How is your eyesight, Corporal?"

"O.K., Doc, sir."

"Do you wear glasses?"

"I lost them in Korea, sir," he drawled.

"You can get another pair before you hit the States. It will take about two weeks before you leave this camp."

"Thank you, sir. Is that all?" he asked.

"Yes." (Maybe he didn't want glasses.)

Two days later he came back.

"Say, Doc," he began, "Come to think of it, I don't see too well."

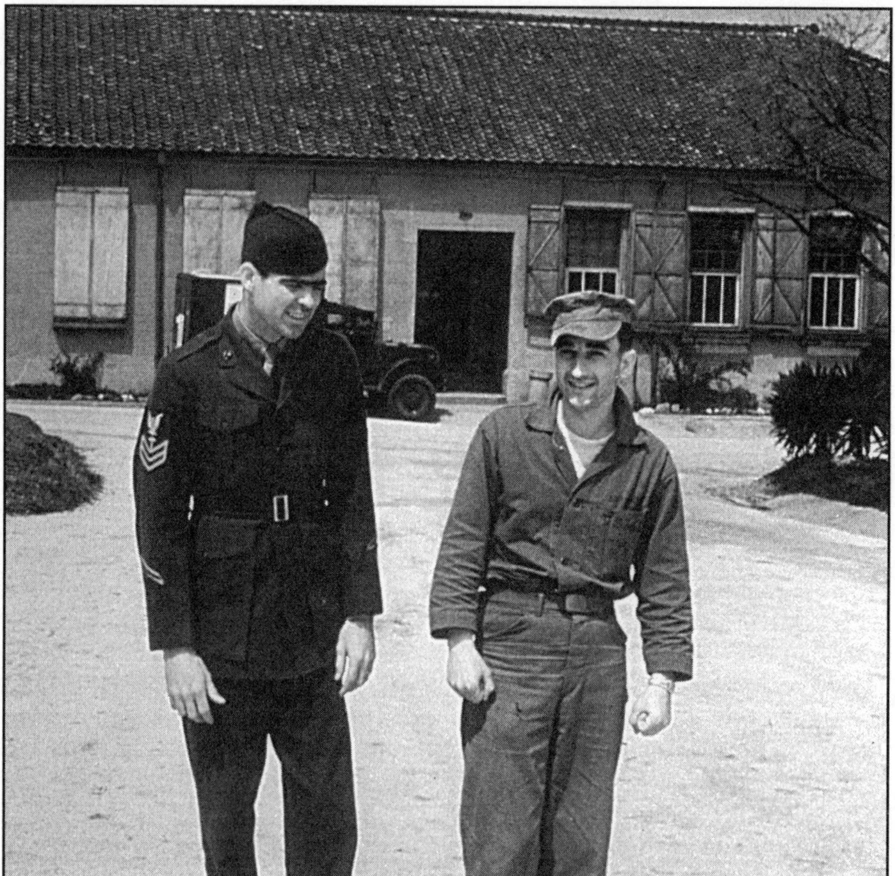

Capshaw and Baird.

"Let me check your vision, Corporal. You stand over there by the door," I instructed, "Cover your left eye and read the chart on the far wall."

"Can't see any letters, Doc, sir."

"Change eyes then," I said.

"Can't see any letters, Doc, sir."

"Both eyes, then,"

"Still can't make any letters out, Doc, sir," he admitted.

I had him move up a bit and he could read some of the larger letters on the top of the chart.

"You need glasses badly," I told him. "I'll send you to the Army hospital. Maybe they can fix you up before it's time to leave Camp Otsu."

Five days later I put in a call for him to report to sick bay to pick up his new glasses. He blossomed out in a big smile as he looked around the room with his new eyes.

"There's one thing I would like to ask you, Corporal," I asked curiously. "How on earth did you ever make out in Korea with that eyesight and no glasses? How could you see to fire a rifle? You were with a squad, weren't you?"

"Yes, sir. I was with a squad," he explained slowly. "I was hopin' you wouldn't ask, but since you have, I guess I'll have to tell you. When we would contact the enemy and the firin' started, I would hit the dirt. When I got organized again, I would look over at the fella next to me, see where he was firin' and point my gun in the same direction. No one ever knew the difference."

All in all, my stay at Camp Otsu was a pure delight - a perfect interlude before returning to the First Marine Division back in Korea.

Chapter Eighteen
VD

As you have undoubtedly surmised by the foregoing, I was not overtaxed by work at Camp Otsu. Soon after my arrival, I made very close friends with two marines. The first was Joe Marini, a man of large stature, in his early thirties and you could tell he was of Italian extraction at first glance from twenty yards away. Joe was the officer in charge of the Mess. He was thus in a position to do me many favors. Joe was a hypochondriac and I was in a position to keep his mind at rest. Joe was a regular marine and had been wounded both in the Second World War and the Korean War. His wounds had healed well and there was no disability.

The second Marine was a tall, thin, intelligent-looking person with a baby face. He was very humorous and often outspoken. Parker was in the Marine Reserve. His wounds made no external marks. Parker never talked about it, but another officer told me that Parker had played a "John Wayne" on top of a knoll with Communist troops coming at him from all sides. Somehow, their bullets and grenade fragments missed him completely as he fought gallantly. One grenade, however, exploded very close above his head and caused internal damage which could not be diagnosed by examination or X-ray. Possibly, we could have visualized his damage today with the advent of the MRI X-ray. For the most part, Parker had no symptoms other than about twice a week he would have a sudden onset of a severe headache. The pain was so severe that he would actually scream with the agony. These headaches lasted only about 15 minutes so there was no need to administer pain medication. The doctors in the navy hospital had put him on Dilantin, but it didn't seem to be doing much for him. Parker was assigned to the motor pool and was a man of leisure, even more so than I.

The three of us were together after working hours each day. Most often we went to the Myaki Hotel in Kyoto for a gourmet meal which cost us fifty cents. This included cocktails and dessert. Together we studied Japanese and Chinese antique block prints, diamonds and pearls. On several occasions, we went to Mikimoto Island and watched the female, topless pearl divers at work. There we learned to classify and grade pearls, and also learned to string pearls. If only we had money to invest. There were 360 yen to dollar. Today 100 yen is worth 97 cents.

One evening, after I had been at Camp Otsu for approximately a month, Parker decided that we should go to Kyoto University and take an evening course in spoken Japanese. We all agreed this was a fine idea and found us a professor that spoke very good English. The professor was very kind to us and spent two hours each evening attempting to teach us spoken Japanese. At the end of a month, our vocabulary was still quite limited, but we understood sentence composition.

Professor Takahashi bowed and said, "If you please, marine officers, you are not going to learn to speak Japanese in this classroom. I wish to introduce you to some Japanese friends of mine who speak fair English and are willing to spend evenings with you."

His technique really worked. We met a number of pleasant, interesting, well-educated and successful Japanese gentlemen who, within another month, had all three of us speaking sufficiently well so that we could converse with the natives. Now you know how I learned to speak limited conversational Japanese, without which I would not have been able to accomplish that which I am about to tell you.

The day after I arrived at Camp Otsu, I became aware that the prevalence of venereal disease posed a gigantic problem for the physician in the Armed Forces.

During my stay in Japan, the prevention and treatment of venereal disease constituted at least 75% of my professional duties and seriously interfered with my quest to learn as much as I could about the Japanese and their culture.

Prior to entering the service, I had seen almost no venereal disease. A general practitioner in a small town in New England very infrequently encounters a case of gonorrhea; a case a syphilis is quite unusual, while chancroid and other forms of venereal disease are unheard of.

On my first day at Camp Otsu, I was conducted on a tour of the sick bay area. The main building was one of typical army barracks construction. One half of this barracks was divided into three rooms: the examination and treatment room, the record department, and the pharmacy. The other half of the long and narrow structure was occupied by offices of the Marine Service Corps Officer and the dentist. A small unmarked corner office caught my eye.

"Is this one vacant?" I asked.

"Hell, no," my tour director replied. "It belongs to the VD contact corpsman. I'll admit he isn't in very often. They keep him on the run most of the time."

"You mean you have a lot of VD in these parts?"

"Are you kidding?" He looked at me closely and decided I wasn't.

"Come out here and let me show you something about what it's like," he offered, motioning me to follow.

The sick bay ward was apart from and at right angles to the main building we had just inspected. As we entered, 22 marines sprang to attention at their bedsides. None of them were bedridden. We made the rounds. One boy had a second degree burn from a Japanese bedwarmer, another was suffering with "back strain", the remaining 20 marines were VD patients.

Back home in New England, venereal disease was still on the "hush hush" list. It was just not proper to go around discussing this topic, especially in mixed company. In Japan, however, I would venture to say that it was a major disease and that it was openly discussed, just as we speak of the common cold orappendicitis.

There were three main sources for contacting venereal disease in the area surrounding Camp Otsu. First, there were the numerous houses of prostitution. They were not outlawed, as is the case in most eastern countries. In one section of Kyoto, our venereal disease contact corpsman counted over 100 such houses. The Japanese public health authorities were obligated to inspect these prostitutes weekly. Actually, this was an impossible task for them. They did not have the properly trained personnel and equipment and money were lacking, as was their technique of examination. An army venereal disease control unit once examined a group of these prostitutes to whom a clean bill of health had been given by the Japanese examiner. The same day, the Army group found 80% of them to be infected with one or more venereal diseases. Another loophole was the reinfection of the prostitutes. A prostitute might be given a clean bill of health, having successfully been treated for a venereal disease. The following day, or even the same day, she might become reinfected. Until this lady of ill repute was examined again, often not for three or four weeks, she was an active carrier of the disease.

The second source of venereal disease contact for the enlisted men was the Cabaret dancers. Since the beginning of the American occupation of Japan in 1946, the number of Cabarets, or nightclubs, had multiplied by the hundreds. A Cabaret was equipped with a bar, dance floor, orchestra, and a floor show. The dancing is conducted quite similarly to that of our "dime-a-dance" clubs. Each evening, selected Japanese girls arrived at the club in evening dress. They had had instruction in the English language and American dance. For the privilege of using the club, each girl paid the management approximately 600 yen (under $2.00). In turn, she made about $1.00 an hour plus tips and a bonus if her customer consumed a large quantity of liquor. As a general rule, it is written in their contracts, or at least there is a verbal agreement, that they were not to carry on with customers after closing hours. In order to avoid trouble with the military authorities, the girls were requested by the management to submit to testing for venereal disease and have a chest X-ray taken for tuberculosis (tuberculosis was very common in Japan at this time). On investigation, however, we found nearly 100% of them were active prostitutes. Most of them were infected with venereal disease. Their fee for the remainder of the night ranged from 1800 to 3600 yen, which was more than most Japanese of the working class at that time made in one month. These fees were easily collected, for by late evening, the male pickups were well-intoxicated.

I will long remember the incident of a contact my corpsman, HM2 Hayden made in a nightspot called "The Blue House." Hayden had complete forms on the girl. He had talked with the manager of The Blue House and had personally asked the girl to report for examination and treatment. We sent a copy of Hayden's report to the Japanese Health Authorities. Three mornings later, Hayden stepped into my office. I was up to my neck with health records at this time.

"Say, Doc, do you remember that contact I made at The Blue House the other day?"

"Yes," I said as my concentration only partially departed from the health record I was working on.

"Well, I went in there last night for a short beer, and who did I see but this same contact we reported last Monday. She is still working. What do we do now?"

"Let's see now," I said looking away from the health record for the first time. "You had better report it to the major's office and ask them to close The Blue House for a few days. The loss of revenue should impress upon them that we are not going to tolerate this type of activity."

The next evening, a marine officer, the chaplain, and I went into town for a movie. On the way home, we decided on a nightcap. Of all the cabarets in town, we had to pick The Blue House. The business of the contact and what I had told Hayden the day before had completely slipped my mind. We had been sitting not more than fifteen minutes and were sipping Asahi beer when the MP's appeared. It was a raid. I tried in vain to talk my way out of the place. They had orders from the major and no one was leaving. Finally, after half an hour, an MP sergeant arrived on the scene and recognized me. We made a hasty departure. I dared not tell my two companions that I had ordered the raid! The next day they came to me with threats of physical violence for someone had spilled the beans.

The third and most virulent source of venereal disease contact is the street walker. I was utterly amazed when I saw the streets literally crawling with these women. We referred to them as "Asiatic Queens". This label had been given to them by the occupational troops. After dark it was not unusual to be accosted by three to five of these "queens" while walking the length of a city block. They made no bones about presenting themselves. I imagine most of them were from the lowest class of Japanese and had been poverty stricken. Even though they had been in the business a number of years, their ability to express themselves in English was quite limited and their approaches were stereotyped.

The usual line for one of these girls was, "you nicea boy. Me numba one girl-san. No BD. You comma with me. OK? Short time treehumbid yen. All night nihumbid yen. OK?"

After being brushed aside, she would give it a second try, thinking she had insulted with a high price.

"How mucha? You speak? Come-a my house. Velly cheap."

If this second attempt failed, she usually retired to a doorway or side alley for they had a deadly fear of the MP's. I was impressed with their knowledge of military information. Certainly, they were organized. It was not unusual to see them leave an area days before the troops themselves moved. Quite often they settled in areas adjacent to a camp site as long as a week before the troops moved in.

I once heard an Army venereal disease control officer make a statement which I am sure is not far from the truth. "One hundred percent of these street walkers are infected with at least one venereal disease."

The queens, of course, have no routine examinations. The best we could do was to have the MP's pick up our contacts and transport them to the local Japanese venereal disease hospital. We were not allowed to examine or treat the Japanese.

The plight of these women was indeed an unhappy one. The war had left the women of Japan with a shortage of men. For many, it was the only way to ward off hunger. In not too many years, however, the memories of the terrible war began to fade and the situation changed. Soon there were signs to show that the Japanese women with their resourcefulness, beauty and their quality of endurance would occupy in the east the position that their American counterparts occupied in the west.

While at Camp Otsu I learned a great deal about the feeling in Japan against the American soldier because of the large number of illegitimate babies born to Japanese women. Most of these children were born to the queens. Even though I lectured and lectured to the men, they did not seem to fear venereal disease. The thought of impregnation did not seem to enter the picture, for if by any chance a queen should make a fuss about being pregnant, an abortion could have been obtained for as little as $4.00. They just would not wear protection.

My lectures to the enlisted men on the subject of venereal disease were at first pathetic. I used medical terms and statistics. It didn't work. As I gazed about the body of troops while spouting medical words and quoting percentages of this and that, all I could see sneers and grins. After a couple of these lectures, I saw the light. Much to the chagrin of the chaplain, I resorted to gory details and the profanity of the enlisted men. These extemporaneous lectures were of some significance in the reduction of venereal disease patients on the ward as long as the interval between them did not exceed one week.

I am sure a short discussion of the various venereal diseases found in the Orient will be of interest to the layman by reason of idle curiosity, if nothing else.

In my small venereal disease ward, the most common disease was chancroid. Chancroid means chancre-like. It was thus named because the sore, or lesion, resembles in appearance the chancre of syphilis. This small oval ulcer is painful, soft, weeping and odoriferous. The true chancre, on the other hand, is painless, firm, not moist and is odorless. It would seem that these two diseases could be easily differentiated clinically. This is not always true, and we must depend upon laboratory procedures. The organism causing chancroid is quite different from that causing the chancre of syphilis. Even though I had made a clinical diagnosis of chancroid, I had a dark field examination performed on the smear. The dark field is a special microscopic method to visualize the organism causing syphilis. We had a number of cases of combined syphilis and chancroid infection. If a dark field had not been done we would have missed the syphilis. The chancre is often overlooked. If this happens it is of tragic consequence, for syphilis then becomes thoroughly established in the blood stream. If untreated, syphilis in advanced stages, can have hundreds of manifestations. In the medical literature it is known as "the great imitator" for it can produce the signs and symptoms of many other diseases.

Chancroid, on the other hand, is limited to the local genital lesion and infection of the lymph glands of the groin. This local ulceration if not treated can become very extensive. While in Japan I learned via the medical grapevine of a case of chancroid in a young serviceman that required amputation and castration. The lymph glands in the groin are enlarged in all cases. If the disease is not treated these glands will often abscess and form draining sinuses.

Gonorrhea, the venereal disease with a score of nicknames in military circles was the second most common. As a rule, this was easily treated with penicillin. It is easily diagnosed by a microscopic examination of the discharge.

A fourth venereal disease had become quite prevalent in Japan. This is called non-specific urethritis. (Gonorrhea is known as specific urethritis.) It is caused by a mixture of bacteria or at least this is what we find on microscopic examination of the discharge. It can cause low backache when the involvement of the prostate is severe.

Where did this fourth disease come from? Many doctors believe it is the result of an inadequate treatment of gonorrhea. I am a firm believer of this theory for two reasons. First, the military services were issuing penicillin tablets as a prophylactic measure to a man going on liberty. One or two of these tablets, in my mind, are just enough to make the gonococcus organism a little sick. The other organisms may then grow readily on the injured tissue.

Secondly, the sale of penicillin was not restricted on the Japanese market. A serviceman may, for a very nominal fee, obtain an injection of penicillin. His purpose in doing this is to keep the listing of a venereal disease from his health record. This one injection is sufficient only to quiet the discharge temporarily. He believes himself to be cured. These other organisms take over and we are presented with another case of non-specific urethritis. I won't go into the present day treatment of this fourth venereal disease, but I will say it is lengthy, uncomfortable, and sometimes unsatisfactory.

Our prize case of venereal disease was a fellow with a "full house", i.e., syphilis, chancroid and gonorrhea all at the same time. If his queen had not been apprehended by my contact man, there would undoubtedly have been others.

When I first arrived at Camp Otsu, the treatment of chancroid was lengthy and rather primitive. As I have mentioned, the disease causes ulcerations on the penis which are very painful. Unfortunately, more than half of the cases of venereal disease were chancroid. Treatment consisted of soaking the penis in a solution of potassium permagnate which is a purple dye solution. Sunlight somehow accentuates the medicinal effect of this dye. Thus, twice a day, when the sun was out, the chancroid victims lined up on the deck of the barracks for a period of soaking followed by lying on their back and exposing their dorcals, as we called them, to the sun. I was often tempted to sneak up and take a picture, but didn't. A few months later, I read in one of our medical journals, that aureomycin (an antibiotic) was effective against chancroid. The Tea Man, our pharmacist, made an ointment of aureomycin by emptying capsules into a beaker containing Vaseline, then mixing the two together. The era of potassium permagnate and purple penises had ended - we had instant cures.

We were required to send a monthly report of our venereal disease census to Tokyo. The reports of our ever-increasing rate of venereal disease reached the Marine Corps commandant's desk. I suspect he was livid, for he wrote a blistering directive to our colonel who in turn called me to his quarters.

"Lieutenant, ah, Doctor, what's the meaning of this outrageous incidence of venereal disease? Can't you control it? My ass is going to be in a sling. I've already got enough troubles. Next, the commandant is going to call me to Tokyo and I am sure you know I already am in deep shit with the Corps." (As I mentioned, the colonel had a bad drinking problem.)

"Yessir, I'll do my best," I assured him.

"See to it!" he bellowed.

"Yessir!" I answered in my best military style. I was sure he was very serious about this.

The following day, I was on the job at daybreak and had all the Corpsmen mustered for plans to reorganize our venereal disease prevention program. I doubled the number of lectures to the troops, pro stations were set up in the surrounding villages as well as additional ones in the Camp Otsu area. VD posters were tacked to all buildings. I borrowed a number of venereal disease movies from a nearby army base. The corpsmen ran these off at every opportunity, with the usual number of faintees. I had several conferences with the Japanese Public Health officials. They agreed to increase efforts to locate and treat contacts. At the end of three weeks, the rate had dropped by 20 percent. I reported this to the Colonel with a resultant pat on the back.

"You're doing a great job, Doc!" he said, then added, "Keep it up!"

No such luck. At the end of the fourth week, the number of venereal disease patients on the ward was within 5 percent of our record census. I responded to another summons from the colonel.

"All right, Doctor, what's the explanation? We were doing fine there for a while. Look at these figures! If you can't do anything about this, I can. From now on, I want to see every marine who is infected with venereal disease, personally. I'll make them sorry they were born males."

"But, colonel..."

"Never mind, Doc, just send me all venereal disease patients."

"Yes, sir."

Within ten days there were no new cases reporting to the sick bay. The Colonel was pleased and told me so. I had no such illusions of grandeur and knew the guys were either getting penicillin from the Japanese market, or were remaining untreated. To prove my point, I made a "short arm" inspection of all hands and sent the report to the colonel's office. The following morning, the colonel did not send for me. He came to my office. His face was crimson red as he burst in with the morning census in his hand.

"Why didn't you tell me this would happen? How was I to know these goofs would pull a thing like this on me?"

"Can't go around telling a colonel how to run his business, sir."

"Well, from now on it's up to you. Do anything, dammit! Get the goddam rate down!"

With this, the colonel stormed out of my office and slammed the door.

"Do anything" the Colonel had said.

These two words kept churning in my head until I had a terrific idea. At last there might be a solution to the venereal disease problem! Within an hour I mustered all of the corpsmen together, including the VD contact corpsmen, behind closed doors. I told them about the colonel being on my back and that this venereal disease problem was really interfering with not only my social life, but theirs. I then told them of my plan and that none of them would be responsible if my plot was uncovered. It was to be my neck and my neck only if the plan fell through.

That afternoon, two corpsmen and I walked to the town of Otsu and visited the public health officials, as well as the local police. Both bowed and agreed to go along with my plan. The next morning I had another meeting with the corpsmen and told them that I needed the assistance of a few MP's. A couple of the corpsmen had MP buddies and agreed to talk with them. They came back and reported to me an hour later.

"Doc, I talked to them and they didn't agree to go along with it, and said you must have holes in your head." They warned, "If you guys get caught, you'll get the axe!"They simmered down a bit after we told them the colonel was in on this, too. "Besides," we added, "you guys will be doing some good for a change. The VD problem has got the colonel down. If he is miserable, the rest of us are going to be miserable." At this point, they agreed to cooperate.

The next evening I took one of my Japanese friends as interpreter and wandered into the district occupied by the houses of ill-repute, even though I thought that I was sufficiently fluent in Japanese by now to do this job alone. We wandered in and out of a number of whorehouses and finally I selected two fairly presentable establishments. We stepped into the vestibule of the first of the two houses, removed our shoes, bowed and asked for the Mamasan. Shortly, the Mamasan appeared and bowed graciously to us. She invited us in for rice, hot sake, and fish. I am sure she suspected that we were there for something other than a visit with one of her girls.

"Tell her why I am here," I said to the interpreter. Mamasan, after hearing the plan, just stood there with her mouth open..

"Tell her it's perfectly legal. She will be running a clean house. Business will boom. No trouble, just yen." It took the interpreter a good ten minutes to convey my thoughts to the Mamasan. She agreed. We had considerable difficulty convincing the Mamasan of the second house until I suggested that we were going to move on to the next establishment and that her business would suffer.

Here's my plan. The girls of these two houses were to report en masse to the Japanese public health department. There they were thoroughly examined and those found to be diseased were immediately discharged by the Mamasan (after being treated by the Japanese). Just to be certain, I gave the girls who had been declared disease-free, a week's course of antibiotic treatment. In addition, they were treated for parasitic intestinal infestations, and instructed as to the proper technique of feminine hygiene which would pretty much eliminate chancroid.

Once this had been accomplished, I rotated the corpsmen through these houses on a daily basis. The MP's on duty saw to it that the marines visited only our private houses. They made it so rough on the street walkers in this area, that they either left town or dropped out of business. I suspect the former rather than the latter. Once a marine entered the house and had taken off his shoes, he was deprived of his billfold by the corpsman, and issued a prophylactic. Before leaving, his billfold was not returned until he had performed a prophylactic treatment. It wasn't long before our venereal disease ward was nearly empty.

At the end of two months, I received a letter from the district medical officer. He wanted to know how I had managed to so drastically reduce the incidence of venereal disease. I never told him. Instead, "...due to extensive lecturing, additional contact work and an increase in the number of prophylactic treatments."

The colonel called me to his office.

"Doc, look at this letter. I don't know how you did it, but I got a commendation from the commandant in Tokyo. Many thanks," he said. "Keep it up."

If he only knew.

It wasn't long before I was on a plane to Pohang-dong, Korea and then on up to the front again - back with an artillery battalion on the western front.

Chapter Nineteen

NEIGHBORLY ASSISTANCE

Midsummer. The pure essence of the word brings to mind fields of flowers, Shakespeare, hot days and endless nights. At least here in Korea two were right. The days of summer were unbelievably hot and the nights were endless. The sound of mortars exploded periodically, their echoes slicing through my mind, invading my dreams.

Chaplain Paul McDowell, Lieutenant Senior Grade, United States Navy was regular Navy and had been in combat with the marines for more than one year. It was midsummer at the time, Mac and I were bunking together in a USMC tent, which was a bit worse for wear. There were dozens of holes in the tent, many of which had been patched, and it still leaked quite badly when it rained. This time of year, however, rain was infrequent. The holes were the result of both artillery shelling and mortar bursts. The dirt floor was packed and swept clean. We had mosquito netting and a tarp set up as a covering for our sleeping bags to divert the raindrops. We both had constructed wooden containers for our rifles, ammunition, 45 automatic pistols, and other gear.

Mac was sitting in a very well-constructed, Korean antique chair which he had confiscated from an abandoned Korean hut. It was too small for him for he was a bit overweight. I was sitting in a large easy chair which I had fashioned from scraps of lumber. The armrests, seat and back were made by weaving strips of rubber inner tubing which I had obtained from the motor pool sergeant. The chair was very comfortable. It was early afternoon and hot, as it usually is this time of year in Western Korea at the 38th parallel. The day had been a quiet one - no casualties and very few sick marines. We were thus taking it easy sipping on a couple of cans of grape juice. The tent flaps were elevated on all sides to pick up any stray breeze. Mac was preparing his sermon for the next morning and I was writing a letter to the folks back home.

Now, I have to tell you a little bit about Mac, or Smiley, as we often called him, who was a fine man of the cloth. He received "rough lip" from the regular marines and went along with their belief that the "Corps" was their Almighty. He rolled well with the punches and he knew well that when they were stressed or wounded, that their religion would somehow become manifest or they would become instant converts. We called him Mac for obvious reasons and Smiley because he wore a grin on his face most of the time. His resemblance to Red Skelton was breathtaking. Mac and I had been together for about two months in Korea and had become close friends.

We had plenty of time to talk and knew quite a bit about each other. One thing bothered me, however. I noticed that he often reached for his crotch as though he were in pain. Finally, I got up enough courage to ask him why he did this. I guess he had been hoping that I'd ask him for he was most anxious to tell me the details of his problem. Mac had not been circumcised as a child and of recent months, the foreskin on his penis had become tight so that it was virtually impossible for him to keep it clean. The medical term for this is phymosis. A low grade infection sets in and the entire end of the penis becomes very tender and painful, especially under the foreskin.

"Mac, the only cure for this condition is a circumcision, and I'm going to have to send you back to a MASH unit to have this done. The colonel will not let me do an elective procedure up here," I explained.

"Come on, Doc! There's no way I'm going to go back to a MASH unit and have all those bastards laughing at me," he argued.

I thought this might be the end of the conversation, but after a few more "Come on, Docs" and several minutes of silence, I gave in and told him that I could do it OK using local anesthesia.

"Gee, Doc, you're a great guy. When can you do it?"

"Well, Mac, I've got to get together the necessary instruments and find a close-mouthed corpsman, either Beauchamp or Rector, to help me. I've got a little something on Beauchamp. I guess I can get him to do it all right and have him keep his mouth shut. Mac, you can't tell anyone about this. I could get into deep shit if any of the brass found out I was doing elective surgery in the vicinity of the front line."

He swore on his Bible that he would tell no one, and I figured that really meant something coming from a Chaplain.

I asked Beauchamp if he would help me with this knowing that he could possibly get into a bit of trouble. He said he was glad to and that Rector would also help us. Beauchamp and Rector, as I mentioned before, were my "personal corpsmen". I called them that for they were assigned to stay at my side at all times in order to make my load lighter and do everything possible to keep me from getting wounded. They were great guys and I often wonder where they are today. They helped me dig my foxholes, made sure I wore my flack jacket (bullet proof vest), that I had enough to eat, and a relatively comfortable place to sleep.

Most of the time I had 30-35 corpsmen under my command. Unfortunately, they were, along with the private first class, the most frequent casualties among the marines. Thus, a large percentage of the corpsmen were either wounded or killed each month and replacements were frequent.

I picked Beauchamp and Rector as my right-hand men. I suspect that they also picked me. I spotted them the day I arrived at the regimental area. They appeared to be opposites, but they were always together. Beauchamp was a tall, young man with blond hair and quite thin. He was a quiet person. Rector was short, stocky but not fat, and had a big mop of dark hair. He was not a quiet person.

The corpsmen call each other by their last names. I tried using their first names, or a nickname, but after a while followed suit. They stayed at my side most of the time and also wore flack jackets. Without doubt they learned a lot of medicine from me during our stay in combat. The three of us became close friends and I also learned much from them.

About a week later, when the enemy had again retreated into their tunnels, Beauchamp, Rector and I cleaned the instruments with alcohol, then

Beauchamp went to fetch the Chaplain. We made sure the other corpsmen were elsewhere. Secrecy was the order of the day. Rector secured the door of the sickbay and I asked Mac to lie down on a cot which we had elevated onto sawhorses to serve as an operating table.

"OK, Mac, take off your pants, get up on the cot and we'll get this over with!" At this point I think Mac was having second thoughts about whether or not he was doing the right thing.

He got a little pale and asked, "Doc, this isn't going to hurt much, is it? Not going to bleed? What's this going to do to my sex life?"

"Come on, Mac. Get up on the cot and forget about sex."

I didn't dare "prep" the end of his penis with alcohol for I'm sure he would have taken off like a jack rabbit in a hawk's shadow. I used some Zephryn solution which we often used to sterilize instruments and prepare the skin prior to surgery.

"Mac, all kidding aside, it's probably going to hurt like hell to put this local anesthetic agent in your penis," I explained, "but after the first injection of novocaine, it shouldn't be too bad."

He didn't say a word.

To my surprise, as I surveyed the instrument tray, I noted an odd looking instrument which I immediately identified as pinking scissors. Pinking scissors are sewing scissors with notched or serrated blades. I remember my mother using them when she was making clothes. They cut the edges of the cloth with a scalloped, or zigzag pattern, which tends to prevent unraveling.

"Rector, where the hell did you ever get these scissors?"

"Doc, I thought these would be great for the Chaplain's circumcision," he answered. Where Rector had found these will always be a mystery to me. I knew it was he rather than Beauchamp.

I showed the scissors to Mac. Much to my surprise he thought it was an OK idea. The pinking scissors were brand new and cut beautifully. The operation went well and we were all impressed with the end result. We told Mac we thought his wife would be quite pleased.

"Mac, you'd better lay low for a few days", I explained, "so that this doesn't get complicated, like infection or bleeding. I'm going to give you a shot of penicillin and tetanus."

Mac got wind on the third day that the colonel was asking about his whereabouts so he surfaced. Actually he was able to walk without the whole thing being obvious by this time. I had told the Colonel that he had a bug and I asked him to stay in his cot for a couple of days.

That afternoon the colonel saw Mac and yelled, "Come on over here, Chaplain! Tell me how you're doing."

Their conversation went well until the colonel looked down at the ground and then for some reason noticed Mac's crotch. Mac had bled a little bit and there was a spot of fresh blood soaking through his pants.

"Damn, Chaplain, have you been hurt or wounded? What the hell's that blood?" he demanded.

Mac broke down and told him the whole story. Fortunately for me, the colonel thought the whole thing was quite humorous, especially when he learned about the pinking scissors.

As Mac and I were sitting in our easy chairs in the tent on that hot afternoon, we didn't have much to do except a bit of writing. Beauchamp and Rector were off getting some grub. Since the day was quiet, I sent the rest of the corpsmen out scouting the area around our present placement looking for North Koreans, who were very adept at sneaking up and cutting our lines of communication. They were quite anxious to do this for a couple of them had recently caught two young North Korean women who had skillfully cut a number of our lines. These were the first women we had seen in nearly a year. Two of the corpsmen were assigned to strip them to make sure that they had no concealed weapons. The North Korean women, after being thoroughly searched, were sent to the rear for interrogation.

We later overheard the men talking, "Man, what figures! I thought all of those gook women were dumpy." After having a couple of fish on the line, they wanted more.

Lippincott, my chief hospital corpsman (HMC), was standing watch in the sickbay tent with which I had a common field phone line. I previously mentioned that the hospital corpsmen are referred to by their last names. This is not to true of an HMC. They answer to "Chief".

My phone rang. I picked up my end of the line just as the Chief picked up his, "Chief Lippincott speaking."

The voice at the other end of the connection was that of a desperate-

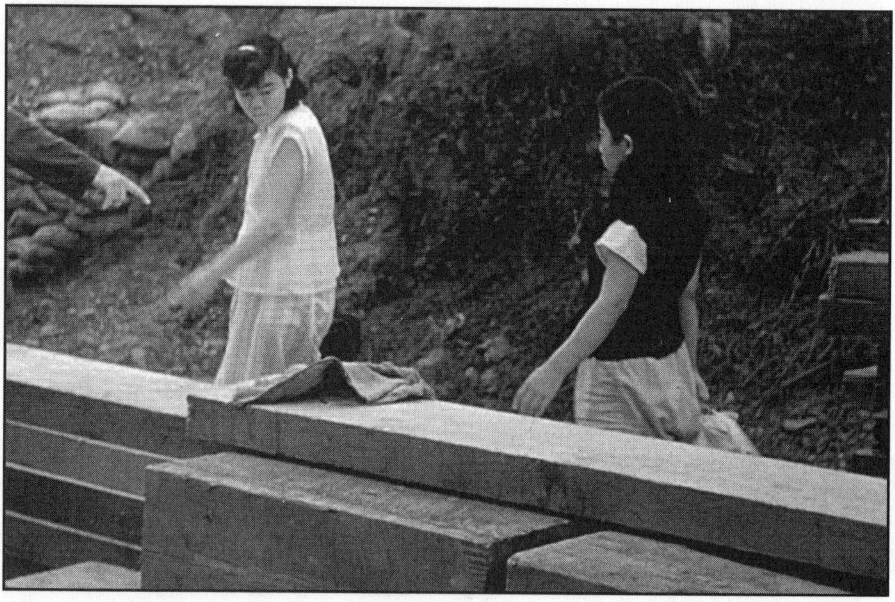

Photograph of two North Korean ladies who were tampering with our communication wires. Little did they know at this point what was in store for them.

ly frightened person. He identified himself as an officer with a moving army artillery battery which was more or less attached to our marine battalion. I guess we needed them because they had some artillery pieces which had a longer range than our 155 howitzers. I'm still not absolutely sure why we needed them. Anyway, our officers directed most of their fire. As a general rule, the marines and army do not mix well. The marines tolerated them by staying away from them. They were referred to as Dogfaces or Grunts. In return, they referred to the marines as Jarheads or Bellhops, Jarhead referring to the marine haircut, and the latter nickname derived from the fact that the dress marine uniform resembled that of a bellhop.

"We're getting hit bad and need medical help! Our medics have been hit! We have no one to give medical aid to the wounded and there are plenty of them! Can you come out and help us, Chief?"

The Chief answered simply, "We'll be right there."

In a couple of minutes the Chief came strolling into the tent - he never did hurry - and was about to give me the message when he saw me picking up my field pack and helmet. At first he said nothing for he knew I had heard the plea for help, then he couldn't resist.

"Hey, Doc. I guess the Dogfaces next door need some help."

Mac said, "I'm coming along with you guys." He knew most of the corpsmen were out. I gladly accepted his offer. Mac was a man of the cloth, but his close association with the sickbay for many months had taught him much about the first aid treatment of the wounded.

I rang the field phone and the colonel answered, "Colonel, I'm going to go next door and give the army guys a hand. I guess they're getting clobbered pretty bad. Beauchamp, Rector, Mac and I are going to take a run over there and see what's going on."

"OK, Doc. I thought I heard some heavy stuff coming in pretty close over to the left. I looked over that way, but I didn't see anything. Why don't you just send some of your corpsmen?"

"They're out checking the lines in the recent vicinity and also getting a breath of fresh air. It was quiet."

"I'll send a couple of scouts out after them. Who's minding the sick bay?" the colonel asked.

"Chief Lippincott."

"OK, good luck, Doc."

On the way to the jeep ambulance we stopped off at the medical supply tent for additional bandages, tourniquets, morphine, plasma, serum albumin, and the like. Beauchamp and Rector checked over the jeep to make sure it was gassed up and was in running order. Then we all scrambled in.

Now, unless you're the driver or on the stretcher, getting into and seated in a jeep ambulance is no easy feat. At first, the jeep ambulance looks just like any ordinary military jeep with a canvas top. The right front and back seats, however, are missing. Along the entire length of the right side of the jeep are two racks which hold stretchers. These can be removed or remain fixed in place. Along the left rear is a metal seat which faces to the right. Thus, any passengers riding in the rear must sit in this very uncomfortable seat facing sideways. There is, of course, no room for a passenger in the front. I took the wheel, for a number of reasons. I was in charge of the mission and thus it was my responsibility. I was in the best position to make snap judgments. Also, the driver's seat was comfortable. No one uttered a word until we had gone about a mile. There were a few groans and moans as we navigated the rough, rutted dirt road with innumerable pot-holes. It was impossible to judge the depth of these potholes because they were filled with water.

Soon, the sound of exploding shells became quite audible off to the left.

"Geesh, listen to that," I said. "What the hell are we getting into?"

There was no answer from the back. My three passengers were pre-occupied trying to stay in their seat. I say seat because they are all facing to the right sitting on the same metal seat. I looked in the rear view mir-ror and could see three unhappy faces and arms stretched out in various directions as they grasped the framework of the jeep.

We came to a point where the road turned sharply to the left. There was also a dip in the road in this area and the road was flooded for a good 20 feet. It was difficult to judge the depth of this water, so I made sure the jeep was in four wheel drive and proceeded at about 5 mph. About halfway through I felt that we were starting to float, so I put the pedal to the metal and made a few waves and splashes. In the summer-time, the side doors on a jeep are removed for better ventilation. We all got splashed.

"Come on, Doc, take it easy!" I finally heard from the rear.

In a few minutes, which seemed like hours, we came to another sharp turn. This time to the right. We were on a summit over-looking the army artillery battery down ahead of us. There was no one in sight. Everything was quiet. Great.

Stopping the jeep, I got out and made a rapid surveillance of the area. Again, I could see no one. My passengers remained where they were. Mac said, "Hey, what's going on?" and then I noticed a few helmeted heads gradually peeking over the edge of foxholes and ditches on the side of the road.

I got back into the jeep and proceeded cautiously down the hill into the artillery area. Then I could see a few men lying in drainage ditches along the road ahead of us. They weren't moving. At that point, a man rose from cover and recognized us as a USMC jeep ambulance.

"Doc! Down there ahead, near the guns! A number of dead, plenty wounded. Some are hurt bad," he yelled. "The gooks got our number and we've been getting clobbered."

We then ducked down as more shells came raining in landing all around the area ahead of us that he had designated. Here we were right out in the open. My first impulse was to turn around and haul ass out of the place in a hurry. After all, this wasn't our job. These guys were Army and not Marine. Also, I was a short-timer. A short-timer is one in combat who has anywhere from a few hours to a couple of months before being rotated away from the combat area. I can remember many a marine corpsman who got it during the last week of combat. Why should I go down there and get my ass blown off? I should have waited for the other corpsmen to get back. This was their job, not mine or the Chaplain's. God, what had I gotten Mac into? I can then remember thinking, "Come on you SOB, these guys are American soldier's and there's only one thing to do, and that's to get down there and get it over with!" I stopped the jeep again and turned to the rear.

"Hey Beauchamp and Rector, you and I will head down there. Mac, this isn't your job, you find a hole and crawl into it and stay there until we come and get you." Mac, looking quite pale, stared me down and shook his head no. I continued, my voice becoming louder with every word, "Mac don't be foolish about this! Get the hell out of this vehicle and take cover!"

Mac continued to stare into my eyes with defiance, slowly his expression changed from open rebellion to mock annoyance and then, enunciating each word for effect, he commented calmly, "That is a hell of a way to talk to a man of the cloth!" He then broke into a big grin.

I pulled the gear down to the left into low and started our descent. The guns were less than 100 yards down directly in front of us. I had the urge to speed up and not be tortured by the long time interval between us and the gun pits. Any speed above 10 mph, however, was out of the question. A wrong turn of the steering wheel would have put us into a muddy rut and this was no place to get out and push. I remember we did have to get out and push at one point.

By the time we arrived at the battery area all was quiet again. We saw no one in the open.

"Geesh, maybe that's the end of it," I remarked almost to myself. No such luck, for just as we pulled up to a couple of bunkers, the shelling started again. We all dove from the jeep for cover. I can just imagine the three of them scrambling out of the end of that jeep.

Beauchamp, Rector and the Chaplain fell into a nice, deep foxhole. I was right next to the entrance of a bunker and dove directly into it from the front seat of the jeep thinking gratefully that I had found the best spot. When the shelling stopped, I lifted my face slowly from the dirt to discover that I was lying in the ammunition bunker! I don't know why, but I laughed.

Suddenly, it was quiet again so I crawled away from my rather precarious location. I looked at the jeep. It had been hit by shrapnel.

The four of us grabbed the medical gear in a hurry and found a large bunker, this time with no ammunition.

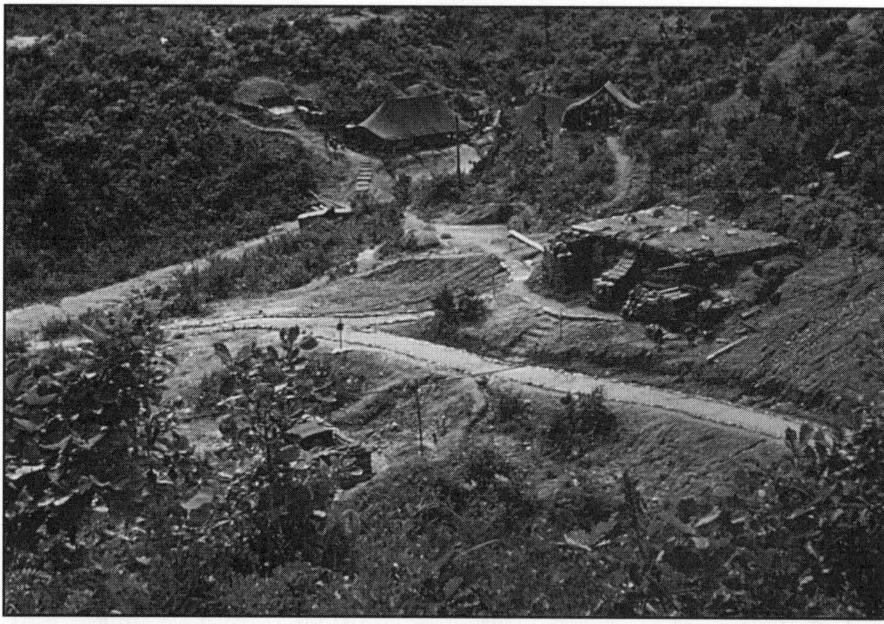

The command bunker for the 11th Artillery Battalion. I later learned that this bunker took a direct hit and all inside were killed.

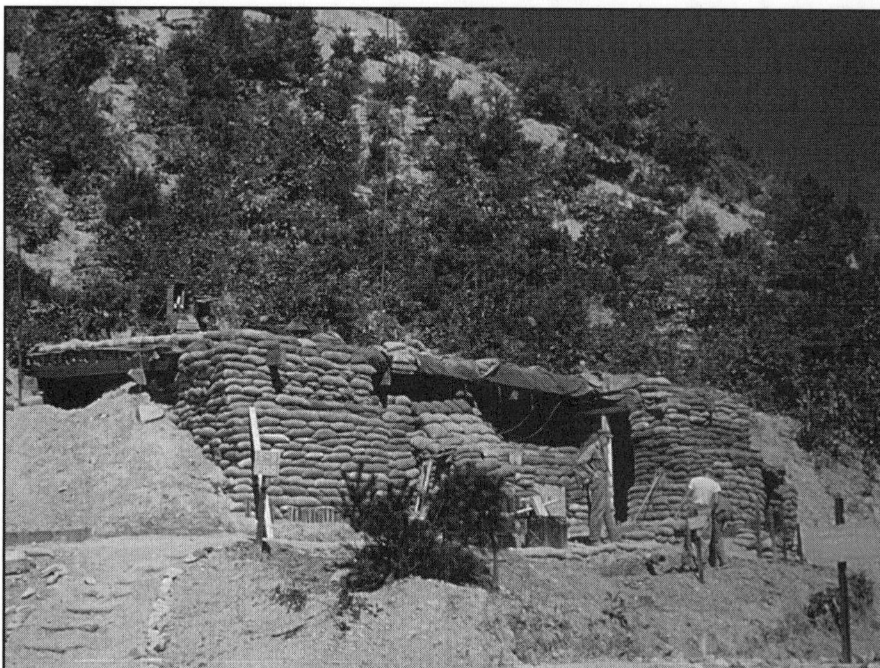

A close-up view of this same bunker.

We had just settled in for a few minutes and arranged out equipment when a dogface sergeant came up on the run,"You guys are medics, right? What do you want me to do?" Now we had a fifth man.

"Where the hell is everybody else?" Beauchamp asked.

The sergeant didn't answer his question, but told us there was a larger and safer bunker right next to us. We all grabbed our medical gear again and crawled after him to the next bunker which was, indeed, quite spacious. There were two soldiers lying inside. The first I examined was very obviously dead. The second was covered with a blanket up to his neck. He was staring with fixed eyes to the sky, for the bunker no longer had a roof.

"You hurt bad, fellow?" I asked. There was no answer. I touched his neck to feel the pulsations of his carotid artery. There were none. He was also dead. I turned down the blanket and saw why. There was a gaping hole in his chest the size of my fist. I looked at his insignia. He was a very young man, one of the battery's medics. He had been caring for the wounded when a large shell fragment came his way.

At this point the enemy shells were again raining in around us. You can't imagine how loud these suckers are and how they shake your very bone marrow. They make Fourth of July fireworks sound like popcorn. I

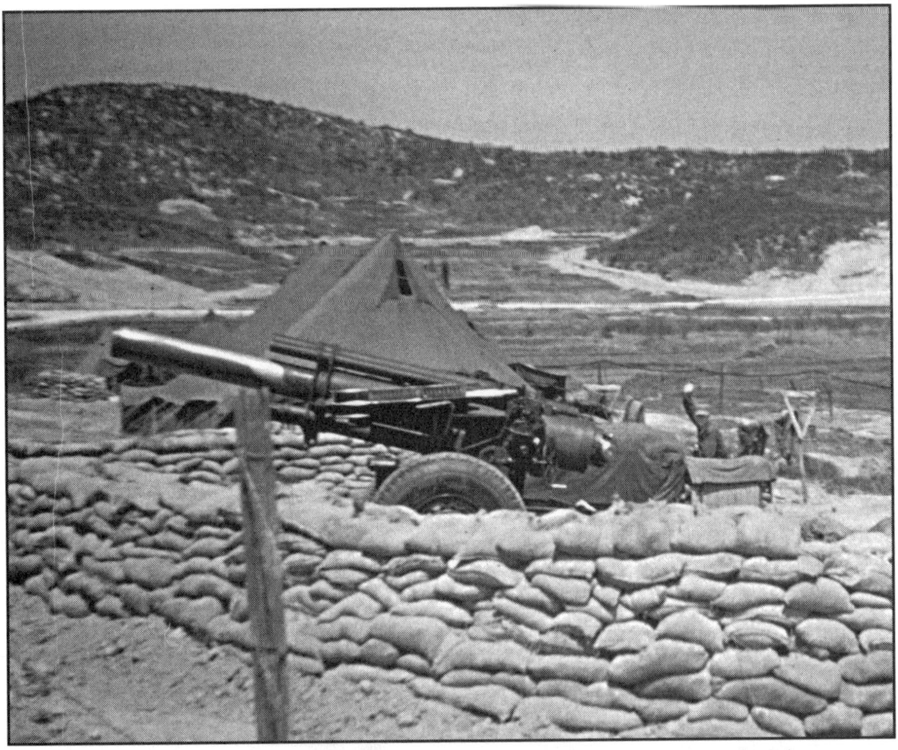

A six inch howitzer with a smoky barrel. The lanyard man is pictured without a helmet. It is impossible to block both ears and pull the lanyard with a helmet on.

looked out the entrance of the bunker and saw a couple of casualties. They were not dead, that is, unless the dead can scream.

We dragged them into the bunker. Beauchamp and Rector had set up ourequipment. I asked the sergeant to get a few of his buddies to drag in some more casualties.

The two casualties on hand were badly hit. The first one who did most of the screaming had a foot missing plus a belly wound. Man, I felt sorry for him and thought if I were similarly wounded that I would probably scream much louder. A tourniquet and dressing to his leg, intravenous serum albumin and a shot of morphine was his treatment for the present time. Rector and the Chaplain had all this done in no time flat.

Beauchamp and I turned to the second. He had been hit with a number of shell fragments. His major wound was to the head. He was only semi-conscious and unable to carry on a conversation with us. We bandaged his head as well as his lesser shrapnel wounds. Since he was not in shock, nor displaying any evidence of pain, I left him for the moment.

The sergeant reappeared with a couple of other soldiers, dragging in two more casualties. The first was dead. The second had multiple shrapnel wounds, none of which were life threatening. Mac and I stopped the bleeding and eased the pain with morphine.

About half an hour passed. Everything seemed to be shipshape in our little "hospital". We carried the three dead soldiers off to the side and concentrated on the two badly wounded ones. We had nine other wounded who were either sitting or lying and in not too bad shape. I studied the two seriously wounded soldiers and decided that they had come to the point where serum albumin and plasma was not enough. They needed whole blood, better treatment than I could give them here in the dirt, and needed it fast.

I looked at Beauchamp, Rector and the Chaplain, "I've got to get these guys to a medical company. The shelling seems to have let up a bit. It's now or never for them. We're not going to get a helicopter in here."

We unhitched the canvas stretchers from the jeep ambulance and brought them to the bunker. We loaded the two seriously wounded soldiers carefully, carried them to the jeep and secured the stretchers in place. I jumped into the jeep. Rector was already in the back with the casualties. As I turned the jeep around and started to drive up the road leaving the battery, the shells were still coming into the area. They were missing the battery completely.

After I had driven a few hundred feet I began to think about where I was and what was happening. Prior to this I had been very busy and everything was sort of mechanical-like. Driving the jeep requires little left brain effort. Again I had the impulse to push the accelerator to the floor and get the hell away. Fortunately, I didn't fall victim to this impulse for we most certainly would have gotten lodged in the mudded rut and there was no way Rector and I could have pushed that vehicle. I guess what kept me going was the frequent screams from the soldier with the amputated foot.

Just as I reached the top of the rise and turned to the left, two army tanks came around the corner and headed down the road towards us. They stopped, blocking our way. I got out and motioned them out of the way, but they didn't move. My choice line of profanity went unheard. The soldier with the amputated foot and belly wound was yelling almost continuously now, even with a half grain of morphine tartrate in his system. He probably needed more at this time, but I was worried about shock.

Suddenly, the tank drivers realized what was going on and literally jumped their vehicles off into the adjacent rice paddy.

I turned the corner into relative safety just as a helicopter appeared from nowhere. He circled above. Evidently someone had put in a call for him. It would have been disastrous for him to fly down into the battery area and he knew it. Both Rector and I got out and tried to motion him to land in the road. He could have easily flown the two wounded men to a medical company in four or five minutes. It would take us at least fifteen, maybe longer. I think he misinterpreted our hand signals, which were undoubtedly wrong in the first place, and disappeared over a hill as our hearts sank.

It was a long trip back to the medical company. The soldier with the bad wound continued to yell and scream with every bump and there were hundreds of them. The head injury case was still quiet. I turned to see how he was doing. He looked dead. Twenty minutes passed before we finally arrived at the medical company. The corpsmen carried the casualties to the receiving tent and the docs set to work on them immediately. They saved both of them.

I glanced over to see Rector dialing the field phone. A relay switchboard produced the same voice that a few hours earlier had called for our assistance. You can imagine our joy when he told us that the shelling had ceased and that Mac and Beauchamp were on their way with the remaining casualties in a "six by truck". We didn't have to go back.

The six by truck made good time and they arrived in about 15 minutes. A few of the casualties were Korean laborers, members of the Korean Service Corps. I spent the rest of the afternoon and evening in the operating tent helping out the docs there. In addition to our casualties from the artillery battery, there were many from a nearby infantry company which had contacted the enemy. Beauchamp, Rector and I scrubbed in and attended to many of the wounded. Mac kept in touch with the army battery by field phone.

One of the wounded Koreans had both hands and feet missing. This was my first and last quadruple amputation. He also had a belly wound. I opened his abdominal cavity and saw his intestines. They were literally filled with large ascaris lumbercoides worms. Two hours of surgery for nothing. He died that night.

Beauchamp and Mac told us that Rector and I had missed the farewell presents from the enemy. A number of shells had landed in the vicinity of the entrance to the battery shortly after our departure. This is where they picked up the South Korean casualties who were hiding in a roadside ditch.

Before crawling into my sleeping bag the next day, I hoofed it over to the colonel's tent to give him a report of my little visit with the army. He provided me with a couple of his straight up martinis, which were much needed, and an interesting epilogue for my story.

At 10 o'clock that evening the army battery received another shower of enemy shells. This time, however, there was no one there. One of our marine patrols had captured a Chinese officer who "obligingly" supplied this bit of enemy schedule. The area had been completely evacuated of men and equipment.

Chapter Twenty

IN MEMORY OF

In a Marine infantry regiment during the Korean War, there are three battalions, and at all times, except during large operations, only two remain active on the front lines, while the third remains a mile or two behind the front for reorganization and rest. The active regiments stay on line for an average of about two months then have a month's reserve. During this month of rest, one afternoon is set aside to remember and pay tribute to the marines who were K.I.A. (killed in action). This is the most impressive military service I have ever witnessed.

A field nestled in a valley under the shadows of the rich green hills adjacent to the marshy rice patties was chosen, leveled by a bulldozer, prepared and stood guard over.

During the morning hours as the golden sun rose in the sky, some of the marines completed the first task in honor of their fallen comrades by filling unused and clean sandbags completely in silence. Each bag was a symbol of the life of a fellow marine that was lost in battle. The sand bags were then carefully squared and placed side by side in two rows, at the head of each a camouflaged helmet was painstakingly placed in tribute.

It wasn't until the sun was beginning to disappear below the horizon that the corpsmen and I began our journey to the cleared field to pay our respects. The long rows of bags seem to stretch out far too long since each bag represented the loss of a human life. My friends and I had started out early. We sat in silence trying to take in all of the men that had been lost when we heard the orderly crunch of marching coming from the other side of the hill.

The marching was slow, even melancholy. Over the crest of the hill a skull and crossbones appeared, the declining sun illuminating it in an eerie glow, setting the mood over the small valley. I knew the writing on the banner before I even read it, "Suicide C". Charlie Company was leading the procession. Charlie Company had a knack for being in the thick of battle and most of the members of the C Company were proud of their nickname which originated from the fact that the company had a hundred and twenty-five percent casualties within a relatively short period of fighting.

Behind, the two other companies followed, led by their company's dog, followed by the buglers, the honor guard, and a small group with musical instruments. In all there were about four hundred. No one uttered a sound as they marched. The dogs didn't bark, the wind didn't blow, the sun didn't seem to move lower in the sky. The only activity was the mournful marching rhythm of the marines' cadence as they approached and took their places.

When the marines were in place, lined up and standing at parade rest, it was as if on cue a helicopter was heard, cresting a hill and touching down. Major-General John T. Seldon stepped out from the aircraft, ducking under the rotating blades, a grim look of sadness set upon his features. As soon as he was clear, he straightened himself, walked briskly to the makeshift podium situated to the left of the officers, one of whom gave a signal for the service to begin.

We snapped to attention and the ceremony began as one of the two buglers sounded church call.

After the small band played the Marine Corps Anthem, the Invocation of prayer was offered by Chaplain Guillaume, a fearless man who had worked beside me on many occasions, who was known and loved by all the men of the battalion, regardless of their faith.

Then Lt. Col. Daughtry introduced General Seldon, the Commanding General of the First Marine Division. General Seldon was a straight-backed marine who outwardly appeared to be a little along in years. A closer look revealed that he indeed was a fairly young man, the careworn expression on his face resulting from the great responsibility of his tour of duty in combat and the ceremony at hand.

The general began slowly and distinctly. His exact words were lost upon the wind, lost as they filtered through to our sorrow filled hearts, but their meaning and essence stayed with me.

"We are assembled here to pay tribute to those proud and heroic Marines of the First Battalion, Seventh Marine Regiment, who gave their lives defending their faith and freedom against the Communist force of aggression from the 10th of March to the 27th of June nineteen hundred and fifty-two. We solemnly dedicate our lives to uphold the torch which they have passed on to us, and we commend their spirits to our Eternal God, who gave them life."

As the general continued, his speech became quite emotional, he wiped his eyes several times and choked on a few words in closing. I am sure he had to cut his speech short. As the National Anthem played, echoing out over the green rice fields, its music drifting higher into the sky over the hills and beyond, I thought of all the marines I had known and lost, not just the ones we were paying tribute to this evening. I felt numb. I knew that numbness was protecting me, like a high castle wall. I never let that wall down. It is the one thing that protects you from going crazy, the one thing that doesn't let you feel too much or think too much about what was going on around you and what had happened to your fallen friends, for if you did, you might not ever return from the chaos of pure madness.

The field fell silent again, and the honors began. Lt. McLaughlin stepped forward to read the roll call of the dead. He took a deep breath and called the first name.

"Staff Sergeant Wayne A. Dykes, Charlie Company."

"Here, Sir!" A voice answered loud and clear. It was the buddy of Sergeant Dykes, who was standing at attention at the head of the first sandbag. After a brief second he sprung into action, raising his rifle over his head and plunging the fixed bayonet into the sandbag. He then picked up the helmet at the head of the sandbag with both hands, placed it on the upright rifle butt and returned to attention.

The roll call of the dead droned on and on. As you hear each name

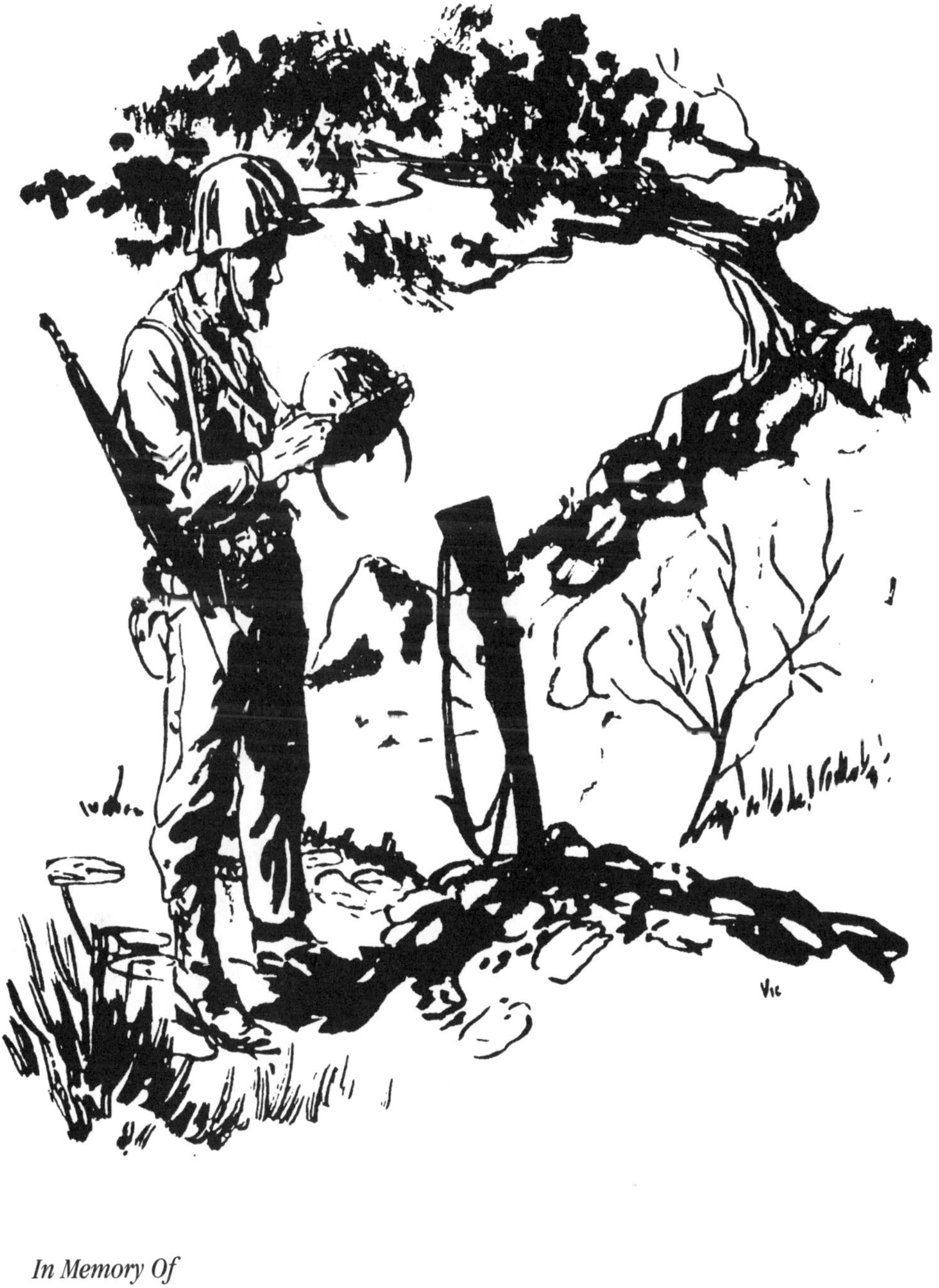

In Memory Of

called you hope, as a chill runs up your spine, that you don't recognize it. The next tribute is called and then the next, its sound hitting me in the pit of my stomach each time. Tom Greene, my friend, was sandbag number three. The wall around me started to crumble, for the first time in combat a tear crept out of my eye. My mind began rapidly to build up that wall again. My eyes dry, the tributes continued and I didn't hear another name uttered.

A well-known, inspiring hymn drifted on the soft blowing breeze. The wind picked up, stirring the valley as if nature was signaling the close of the solemn service.

An Honor Guard then fired the rifle salute as the sun finally fell beneath the hills. The bugle sounded, its echo fading into the chaplain's closing prayer and a benediction.

The cleared field with its two rows of sandbags, rifles, and helmets stood in still, majestic, silence flooded with the blood-red glow of the setting sun.

As we slowly walked back to the camp area, we dared not to talk for fear of breaking down and showing how we really felt - like crying.

Chapter Twenty One

DEPARTING

It was October, 1952, finally time for me to leave the MLR and return home. Many of us who were leaving didn't talk much about it for fear of jinxing it. We worried that the enemy would launch a push in a southerly direction and we would end up one of those unfortunates who get hit during the last few days of combat. I was to leave with a few other officers and enlisted men. None of us showed much emotion and the goodbyes were all short. Departing the friends I had been with in combat for so long left me with a deep sadness.There would always be a bond with my fellow marines. The friendships you make in combat never leave you, but, on the other hand, they often never survive outside of this war torn environment.

I especially hated to leave our little dog "Georgie", who was a survivor if I ever saw one. He had somehow escaped from being the main course on a hungry Korean dinner table and had also survived the artillery and mortar shellings. My mind, troubled and saddened, was anchored in emotions, but my heart was soaring. I was going home.

We departed from the combat zone with several vehicles in our convoy.Without fail the enemy intelligence was excellent and the gooks gave us a send off that splintered the sky with a few rounds of artillery shells, luckily never coming within three hundred yards of us. I had said my goodbyes back at the Battalion. I was already out of Korea, my mind traveling ahead as if to lead the way.

I abruptly, and reluctantly, came back to the present when we arrived in Sasabo, Japan. Here officers and enlisted men were advised to form a line to be tested for malaria in one area, deloused in the second, and to be given medication for intestinal worms in the third.The kidding around by the jokers made an unbearable situation tolerable.We even attempted to estimate the number of dead worms that had entered the Sasabo sewer system as a result of our presence.

The next day, I was even more excited to be going home, as we marched in formation in Marine Corps fashion to the troop ship which was a merchant marine affair with a ten degree list. It size was overwhelming, it was a truly awesome sight. Much to my surprise there was a large number of army troops waiting to return to the States aboard the ship. I soon learned that these men were for the most part rear end pogues who had not been in combat. As soon as I saw them I knew we were in for a bit of trouble on the trip back to civilization. Marine and army personnel as a rule do not amalgamate. The volatile situation was readily taken care of by the quick action of some alert officers in both branches and the worst injury was to some pride and egos due to some isolated name calling.

The army and the marine troops were separated to different decks of the ship. I bunked with a few other officers on the second deck way up near the bow on the starboard side. Gratefully I got the top bunk, preferring to look at the bulkhead, rather the underside of another bunk.

Lights were out at 10 p.m. The ship was tied to the dock at Sasabo,

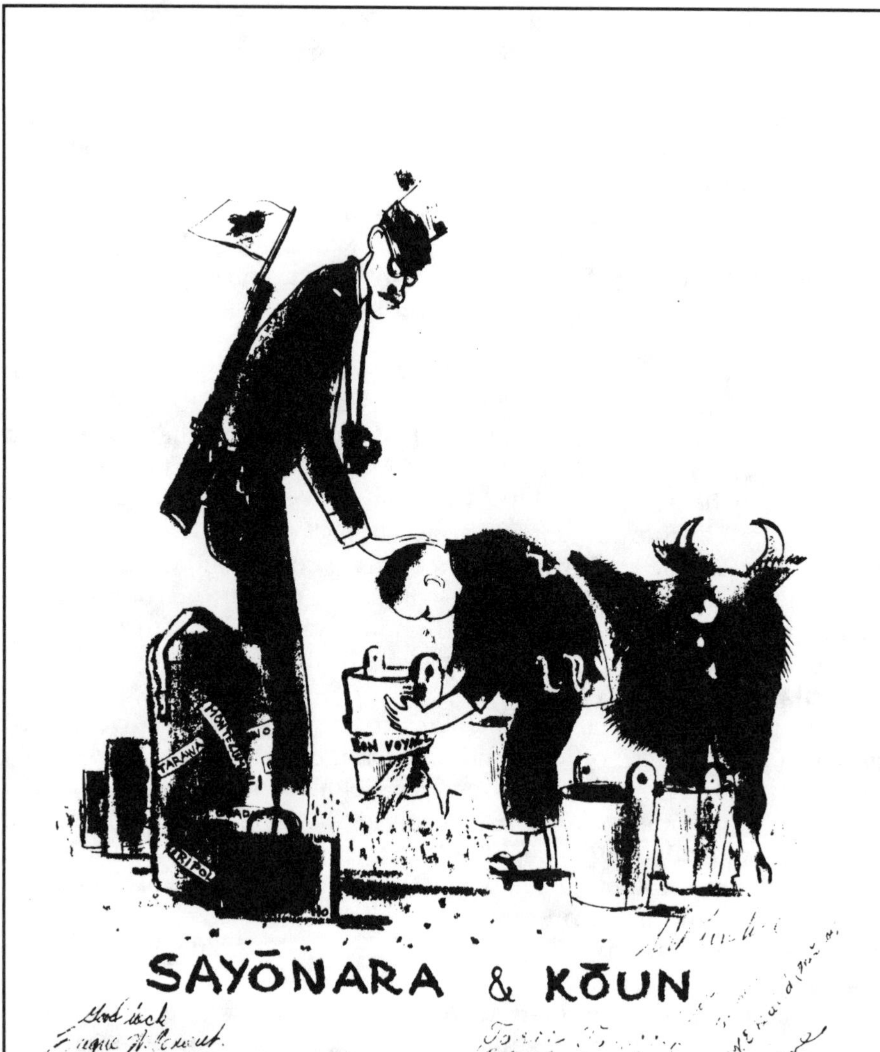

"Good-bye and Good Luck"

swaying slightly with the movement of the water. This motion, along with studying the construction of the bulkhead was quite conducive to sleep and my conversations with the other officers was short-lived.

I awoke the next morning feeling more refreshed than I had been in months. I dressed quickly and ran out to the railing. We had left the dock and were far out at sea, there was no land in sight. What a strange feeling not to see any form of land. We were completely isolated on a floating island, or a city at sea. The next five days seemed to pass as if in a pleasant dream. I met the medical officer and corpsmen of the ship, we talked, ate, drank, and played cribbage.

On the fifth day, the mood of the dream shifted in to that of a minor nightmare. The blue sky had disappeared and the wind began blowing fiercely and the sea became uncomfortably rough. Over the loud speaker they warned us we were heading into a typhoon and we were advised to hold on to the railings and to make sure the straps were firmly in place when we were in our bunks. What? Shouldn't we avoid going into a typhoon? Most of us were landlubbers and seasickness increased to epidemic proportions. There was vomit everywhere, the smell invaded every corner of the ship. There was no escape even on deck in the wind and pouring rain. The mess hall was empty with the exception of some of the ship's crew. I, fortunately, did not get seasick, but limited my activities and intake to an occasional cup of coffee. We attempted to play cribbage, but this was not possible. If you let go of your coffee cup for a split second, it skidded across the table onto the deck.

The storm continued for two more days and I resigned to pass the time reading inside my cabin, strapped into my bunk. I was reading there on the third day of the storm when the ship's doctor, George, came in looking a little concerned.

"Hey, Monty! I think I we have a medical problem. There is a dogface down in sickbay who has a fever, elevated white blood count, and all the classic symptoms of acute appendicitis, in addition to his seasickness. This soldier is in bad shape. I was hoping you could come down and take a look at him with me." At this point he nearly went on his ass as the ship hit the peak of a pitch and began to roll.

I agreed, unstrapped myself from the bunk, crawled down in between the pitches of the ship and we staggered down to the sick bay. We found the army enlisted man, named Edward, lying in a bunk covered in vomit and moaning. To say he looked real bad was a gross understatement. The soldier stopped moaning and in a voice as quiet as a whisper, laced with a undercurrent of intense pain he spoke to me.

"Come on, Doc, I'm dying. You've got to do something! My gut is on fire!!"

I nodded and felt his abdomen. There was no doubt in my mind concerning his appendix. It was red hot and had to come out. I turned to George and nodded yes.

George then leaned down and told Edward that the operation was imperative. Edward said, in between moans, he didn't care what we did, just as long as we got the pain to stop.

Three of the corpsmen placed him on a stretcher and carried him to the operating room. It took us at least ten minutes to strap him to the operating table. He didn't want to be strapped down. I wouldn't have either. He was thrashing around in agony and occasionally wretched with the dry heaves. Our moving environment didn't make things any easier. The shot of morphine and atropine finally took effect and he calmed down sufficiently so that we could secure the straps. Actually, he was becoming quite euphoric.

Getting the instruments together was no easy task, either. First we tried a regular Mayo stand, which was taped to the deck, and this didn't work. One of the corpsmen who had been at sea a few times fashioned a basket from sheeting so that the instruments wouldn't be thrown into one another and onto the deck.

"George, I'll give anesthesia and you do the operation," I suggested.

"No, Monty. You do the operation and I'll give the anesthesia. I haven't done an appendix in quite a while."

"Neither have I, George. You're the ship's doctor, you should do the surgery."

"OK...I guess I'm up to it."

"What do you have for anesthesia, George? There is no way we can give him spinal anesthesia safely with all this motion!"

"I guess it will have to be open drop ether, Monty."

I placed the ether mask over Edward's face and poured a couple of drops from the ether can. He didn't seem to mind it. Ether in small concentration has a not unpleasant odor. As it becomes more concentrated, the odor is very offensive, then is followed by a stage of excitement, anxiety and fright. Edward passed through this stage rapidly and was soon unconscious.

We had intravenous fluids flowing into his veins to counteract his dehydration. George prepared his belly with an antiseptic solution and started the operation with two corpsmen.

Watching the three of them, I was somehow reminded of people trying to stand in a bus traveling over a rough road. After a while George got the hang of it and would operate only when the ship peaked in a roll or pitch.

Their scrubbing before the operation was quite limited. They wore only cap, mask and gloves during the surgery. The field was draped with four towels and a half sheet. The half sheet was a farce and was soon on the deck.

"Hey, Monty! How is the anesthesia going?"

"Fine, George."

"How about coming down here and giving me a hand. One of the corpsmen can continue with the anesthesia."

Both corpsmen thought this was a bad plan.

"We don't know how to give anesthesia!"

"Come on, you guys. There's nothing to it. All you have to do is hold the mask over his face and drip ether with the other hand when we tell you. Put your fingers under the chin like Monty's doing...lift up the chin."

One of the corpsmen took my place and the second continued to hold the retractors.

George and I, after some time, were able to extract the appendix, which was indeed acutely inflamed, but not ruptured. I suspect his scar was not the best in the world. At least the skin edges were approximated. As luck would have it, he never turned a hair and there were no postoperative complications.

The storm ended the next day. The night before, I had a nightmare. I dreamt I was home in Vermont. Three children were playing in my room and had found my 45 automatic pistol. One child was shot and severely wounded. This dream was so vivid, I can still remember it after all these years.

I unstrapped myself from the bunk, sat up in a cold sweat, shook my head and jumped down to the deck.

Someone said, "Where are you going, Monty?"

"Go back to sleep," I answered quietly.

Fumbling around in my duffel bag, I found my 45 in its holster attached to a webbed belt. It had beautiful handcarved pistol grips and an extra new barrel and a hand tooled leather holster. I staggered out to the deck and stood there a minute hanging on to the railing, going over my dream.

The stern of the ship was going up and down like a fast elevator in a 6 story building. When the stern hit the bottom of a trough, it was quiet

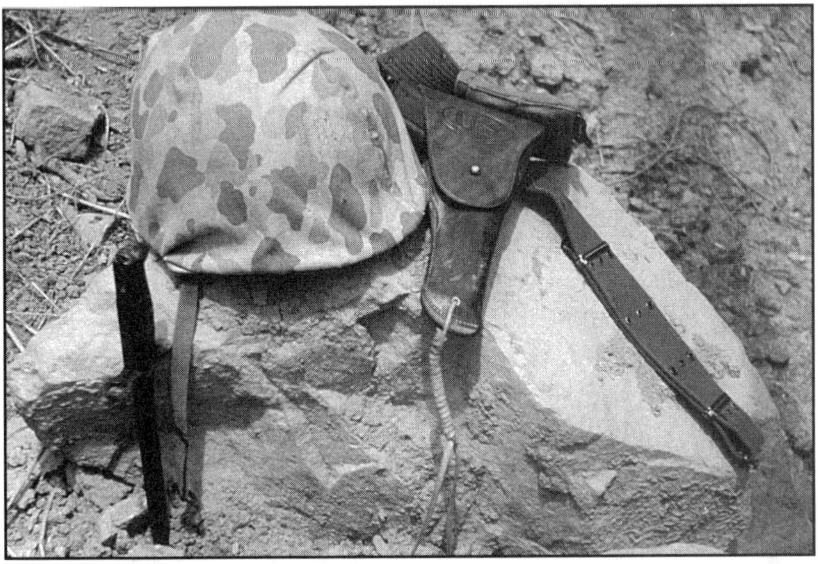

A still life of my bayonet, helmet and 45 automatic.

for an instant for the next splash on the deck had not begun.

Over the side went everything but the webbed belt, which I still have today. It is my only material link to combat in Korea. Would the dream have come true?

After 23 days at sea, we passed under the Golden Gate Bridge in San Francisco. There was a band playing The Marine Corps Hymn, and a couple of beautiful vocalists. I never did get their names. I had only one thing on my mind, and that was a fresh glass of milk! In the early 50's it was impossible to obtain fresh milk in either Korea or Japan. It didn't take me long to find a grocery store and purchase a quart of homogenized whole milk. I deposited the empty container in the trash barrel on my way out of the store.

Soon I would be back in New England, embraced once again by my family, friends and neighbors. I would be able to see the magnificent fall foliage of my hometown in October, a most beautiful time of year in Vermont.

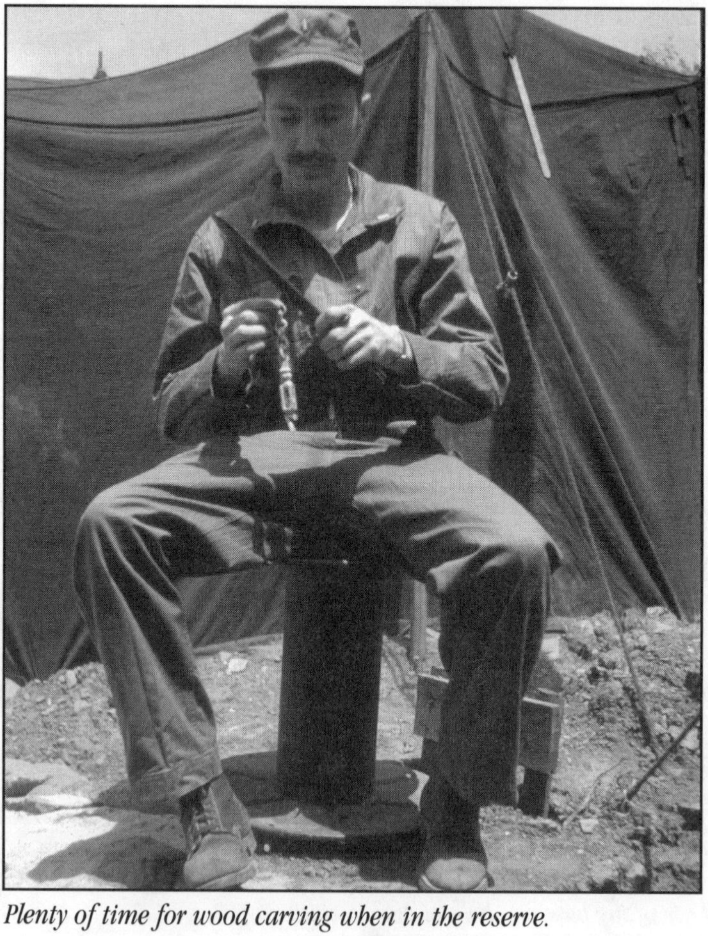

Plenty of time for wood carving when in the reserve.

I knew I would forever think of the war in Korea where I watched men die, where I repaired the wounded - both friend and foe. I left the combat situation with the thought that I had survived any physical and, for the most part, mental trauma. All this changed me and I'm not sure how. It was a change that never left. It certainly taught me some of the most crucial lessons of my life.

I discovered how to accomplish as much as possible with my time, getting the most out of the time you have in each day, to be thankful for being alive and to appreciate the joys, and cope with the sorrows of life. I learned to be tolerant of myself and others, and not to hate anyone or anything. Most of all, I learned how to control my emotions and be able to forget that which needs to be forgotten. I never really hated the enemy like I was supposed to, for somehow I knew they were people like us from a different culture, but with families back home.

I learned how to be a marine. They taught me how to survive in the outdoors in a frigid climate and in tropical weather. I learned how to fire a 45 automatic pistol, carbine rifle, throw grenades, fire a bazooka, and a 155 howitzer. All these things I could do, but I skillfully avoided the BAR (Browning automatic rifle) after firing one once. I also learned how to dig foxholes, build bunkers both with sandbags and into the side of a hill and to live on canned food.

I learned to do many surgical operations I had never performed previously, on the American, North Korean and Chinese wounded. I learned to diagnose and treat tropical diseases and live with rats, snakes and insects. I learned how to gather information.

One thing is certain. I learned that war is futile. No one ever wins, except perhaps for the politicians and the people who manufacture combat equipment.

There is a big difference between the regular and reserve marine. The regular marine is a professional soldier. The rest of us were from the Marine Reserves, or had been drafted and transferred to the Marine Corps, either voluntarily or involuntarily. You can spot a regular marine anywhere. They stand straight, are always well-dressed even in combat, neat and clean. To put it in one context, the Marine Corps is their religion and they follow this religion just as a Jesuit priest or a Buddhist monk does his.

Throughout my experience in combat, I continued my wood carving. In Japan I had brought a jackknife that had four wood carving tools instead of blades. My best piece during the Korean war was a letter opener which extended into a chain and a ball within a cage, all carved from one piece of wood. I had the "First Marine Division" carved into the handle. It's now in the hands of the marine officer who admired it and offered to buy it except he didn't have any money. Most of us didn't. I wouldn't have charged him anyway. Unfortunately, his name escapes me, but I'll bet he still has it among his war mementos. Maybe he will read this and let me know.

Epilogue

Much of my life since returning home from Korea has been involved with teaching Harvard Medical students and doctors training to be specialists, examining and treating patients in an office setting, performing surgery, and finally, research. All of this has been very gratifying. I have learned that the greatest satisfaction in life is what you can accomplish and what you can do for others.